How Generosity Works

The Intention to Benefit Others

Janet Kathleen Ettele

DIAMOND CUTTER PRESS

Published in 2011 by Diamond Cutter Press

Book design by Clare Cerullo

Printed in the United States of America

Library of Congress Cataloging-in-Publication Data is available upon request.

ISBN 978-0-9765469-8-6

www.diamondcutterpress.com

This book is dedicated with love and gratitude
to the patient and kind monks
who have been my teachers
and who demonstrate the way of the Bodhisattva
through all that they do.

Introduction

A Guide to the Bodhisattva's Way of Life (Bodhichayavatara) was first taught by Master Shantideva in India during the eighth century. He was born a prince, but chose the life of a monk and studied at Nalanda University. While at Nalanda, Master Shantideva appeared to do nothing but sleep, eat, and other necessary functions of the body and was perceived by the other monks to be an embarrassment to their prestigious university. The monks resented him for his laziness, and since there were rules that prevented them from having him expelled, they designed a plan they believed would be a perfect way to shame him into voluntarily leaving Nalanda. The plan included ordering him to give a public teaching. They thought that certainly he would realize that since he knew nothing and had nothing of value to teach, he would run away to avoid humiliation.

In the center of a field, they prepared a very high throne for him to teach from and invited people from all the surrounding areas to attend. To increase the challenge, they asked him to teach something that had never been taught before. Determined to leave no stone unturned in their effort to humiliate him, they had built the throne with no stairs by which to reach its seat. When Shantideva approached the throne, he placed his hand on its side and was immediately transported to the seat of the throne. Then, Shantideva proceeded to speak eloquently and spontaneously, reciting the Bodhichayavatara, which is now one of the most renowned texts in Buddhism. To the astonishment of those in attendance, the profound teaching flowed from Shantideva in the form of song-like poetry. It has been said that when Master Shantideva reached the final chapter on the Perfection of Wisdom, that his body raised higher and higher from the seat of the throne until he eventually disappeared from sight. His teachings continued, but his voice could only be heard by those who, having attained higher realizations in their own minds, had the ability to hear them.

A Guide to the Bodhisattva's Way of Life has provided students of the Buddhist Dharma from that day forward with what is commonly known as the Six Paramitas, or the Six Perfections. The Six Perfections provide the necessary guidance on how a Bodhisattva, motivated by compassion and the intention to benefit all beings, must perfect his or her mind on the path to enlightenment. For ordinary people like most of us, the verses provide the perfect guidance to live happy and meaningful lives.

The first of Master Shantideva's Six Perfections is the Perfection of Generosity. This perfection teaches us about unconditional love, and about giving compassionately without attachment or expectation. It also illuminates the most generous motivation—the motivation that is free from discrimination, and carries the intention to benefit others.

How Generosity Works is a story that threads Shantideva's verses from "The Perfection of Generosity" into a contemporary setting of ordinary people living ordinary lives. It is my deepest hope that this story will illustrate the timeless value of Master Shantideva's teachings and will serve to "plant the seeds" for happiness and true peace for all sentient beings.

Part
One

Lessons

This intention to benefit all beings,
Which does not arise in others even for their own sake,
Is an extraordinary jewel of the mind,
And its birth is an unprecedented wonder.
I. v. 25

It was a day that began like any other—when waking up happens only after sitting up and planting feet on the floor. January mornings are always cold in New England, and the early light washes the world in colors of grey violet. Grace sat on the edge of her bed, taking in the sounds of the house—the hum of the old refrigerator, a clock ticking in the next room, and then, a bird singing in the bitter cold outside the frost covered window. She was inspired by the song—full of joy and courage in the face of icy cold.

Life had changed for Grace in a way that felt abrupt although in truth was gradual in its arrival. The hectic morning routine of gathering her sons together and delivering them to school before the tardy bell rang had been replaced by solitude and quiet. With the boys grown and no longer living at home, Grace felt the strange phenomenon of time collapsing within a heartbeat while clearly reflected in the older face that greeted her in the mirror. The light caught strands of silver hair growing from her center part, and she wondered if this new look might pass for professionally done blonde highlights since things like hair coloring and manicures aren't included in a tight budget. Shaking off the downward spiral that thoughts of vanity, aging, and fiscal disaster invite, she pulled a sweater over her head and thick wool socks on her feet, and walked downstairs to the wood stove. The embers still glowing from the night before ignited the crumpled pieces of newspaper and kindling that she fed the stove. Letting it crackle and blaze before adding a heavier log, she left the stove door open just enough so the draft could work its magic on the flames, and soon the house would be warm.

In the dim light that spilled from the fire, the baby grand piano caught her attention. Its top was propped open and the keys had the appearance of crushed velvet in the morning greyness. The piano consumed a lot of space in her small home. On this particular morning, she stopped and watched it as if looking for signs of life. She was reminded of her father and smiled in appreciation of how, in his own gruff way, he had supported her interest in music. Grace's younger dream to be a composer was replaced by teaching. She grew to love the students that came for their piano lessons and the liveliness they brought into her home.

Morning routines cushion the day's entry, and Grace savored this ritualistic part of her day. It was too early for the phone to ring, and the stillness and silence had a sacred quality. Filling the coffee pot with water, measuring the coffee in scoopfuls, assembling the percolator, and setting it on the stove was so well rehearsed, it could have been done with eyes closed. While the routines of building the fire and preparing the coffee filled the house with warmth and wonderful smells, it was her daily practice of meditation that provided the sweetener.

Several years earlier, an unplanned stop on a Saturday outing changed the path of Grace's life. Some of life's most interesting relationships are the most unlikely and least expected. And some of the most significant and pivotal encounters are those that happen as if by chance. Grace felt these experiences reveal evidence that magic intersects with the mundane. They carry us to the threshold of transformation if we choose to pursue them. The day a particular book caught her attention as she rummaged through the discounted shelf in a bookstore was one of those transformational moments.

It was an October afternoon with an azure sky that postcards are made from, drenched in sunlight, and bordered by trees whose leaves were in their peak of autumn red, gold, and orange. The sun felt good warming her back through her jacket, and the bookshelf outside the store gave her an excuse to soak in the sun's warmth. She shuffled through the assortment of cookbooks, books on travel, how-to-books for achieving the perfect body and then, a thick hardcover book with an appealing cover. There was something about the graceful serenity of the Buddha's statue seated in the Zen garden that compelled her to take the book from the shelf. Flipping through its pages, glancing at chapter headings and photographs, she stopped on one page where she read, *"The Buddha said, 'My teachings are a finger pointing to the moon. Do not get caught in thinking that the finger is the moon. It is because of the finger that you can see the moon.'"*

The poetry of this phrase had a simple and eloquent wisdom that resonated for Grace. She had an interest in various spiritual traditions, and Buddhism was one she knew very little about. In this case, she wasn't sure what the moon might offer, but the passage felt like an invitation to explore the Buddha's teachings with a questioning mind. Even if it were simply to expose herself to another philosophical view of life, the humbleness of the invitation aroused her curiosity. She held the book while she evaluated buying something that wasn't a necessity. When she saw the sales price was a good one, her decision was made, and she entered the store to pay the cashier.

⌣

How can I fathom the depths
Of the goodness of this jewel of the mind
The panacea that relieves the world of pain
And is the source of all its joy?
I. v. 26

The Buddha sitting in the Zen garden was her companion at breakfast, dinner, bedtime, and any other time when there wasn't a demand for her attention. Dust gathered a little more heavily on furniture and in the corners of the baseboards, mail accumulated and remained unopened a little too long, and trips to the grocery store were contingent on whether or not there was enough coffee and cream for the next morning. Many times, invitations from friends were politely declined. Even when she wasn't reading or trying her hand at meditation, the thoughts presented in the book had a way of blending with the activities of her day. Preparing meals became a meditation on gratitude, and sitting in traffic became an opportunity to wish happiness to all who were on the road with her. Over time, a fledgling collection of Buddhist teachings grew into several towers of books that formed on end tables, coffee tables, and nightstands. With each new level of understanding, new questions came to mind that she wanted answers to, and so one book led to another that led to another, and so on.

One day, while driving on a road she had driven on for years, she saw something she hadn't noticed before. Tibetan Prayer Flags were strung from trees that flanked a stone-covered driveway, and there was a small sign for a Tibetan Buddhist Teaching Center. The old Buddhist proverb, "When the student is ready, the master appears," echoed its truth in this moment. She turned her car around and coasted down the slope of the bumpy driveway. Noticing other cars in the small parking area, Grace was hopeful there would be someone there who could give her information about classes.

The sign on the door invited visitors to enter during their posted hours. Grace checked her watch and opened the door. The center looked like an old farmhouse, and once inside, she felt as if she had just entered someone's home.

"Hello?" She stood in the foyer, unsure of where to go.

She heard a deep voice answer, "Hello." A man came from the next room wearing black-rimmed glasses, jeans, and a blue buttondown shirt. "I'm Ned," he said. "Welcome. Please come in."

"Thank you." She reached out to shake Ned's hand. "My name is Grace."

There was a row of shoes and boots on a rack by the front door. Seeing that Ned was wearing socks, she removed her shoes and placed them near the others. Ned led her to a room where there was a large table with books and papers spread over its surface. Windows offered a view of gently sloping lawns, gravel walkways, and a pond that was fed by a rock lined stream.

"Have you been here before?" Ned asked.

"No," she answered. "I just noticed the sign out front that says this is a teaching center, and I'm interested to know about the classes."

Ned gave Grace a schedule of classes with a brief description of each one. He explained that they were taught either by Rinpoche or Geshe, two of the monks who lived at the center, or by other monks who visited. He showed her the Gompa where classes were held. Its walls were decorated with paintings on cloth depicting the life of the Buddha. Tables covered with flowers in vases, lit candles, and small glass containers filled with yellow saffron water surrounded a bronze statue of Buddha. Ned was an enthusiastic tour guide, answering questions Grace asked and even more that she hadn't asked. He invited her to attend any of the classes and reassured her that it didn't matter whether or not she was a Buddhist. There were things she could learn that would be quite applicable to daily life situations.

Grace began attending classes and found that the material she had studied in books was enhanced by the instruction and guidance of the monks. The meditation practice she wrestled with began to soften into a calm, focused state of mindfulness. When she first heard Rinpoche teach, she listened spellbound. He taught from texts that he knew so well that the words flowed with the ease that someone might rattle off a favorite recipe they had committed to memory. After a few years of listening, studying, and putting into practice all that she was learning, she gradually began to view life and its circumstances through a different lens. She learned to respond to things more calmly and with a deeper awareness. She began to fully appreciate that, in Rinpoche, she had found a genuine guide who had all the earmarks of someone she could trust to teach with the perfect balance of compassion and wisdom. It also prepared Grace for another unexpected meeting on the icy-cold day in January when our story begins.

⌒

Although wishing to be rid of misery,
They run towards misery itself.
Although wishing to have happiness,
Like an enemy they ignorantly destroy it.
I. v. 28

The answering machine was doing its job when Grace walked into her house. She stood in the front hallway and listened to the message while she stomped the snow off her boots and took off her coat.

"Hi, Grace, it's Maureen Reilly. I just wanted to give you the heads up that I can't take Natalie to her lesson today. Brian's son is home from college, so he'll be taking her for me. I've asked him to wait there while Natalie has her lesson. I hope that's okay with you. G'bye."

Hearing this message was a relief. Maureen's nervous energy was so high that Grace could feel the tension when she approached the house, jabbering instructions at Natalie. It often took a little preparation to greet her warmly. Grace would begin by closing her eyes, then taking a few breaths to open her heart before Maureen walked through the door. Inevitably, Maureen would purge every activity and event of her week with martyr-like importance. Her list of problems included things like arranging delivery for the living room set she had just ordered, or choosing the right knobs for her new kitchen cupboards. Everything was burdensome and complicated for Maureen. Her attitude towards Brian's children from his first marriage was, like most everything else, unpleasant.

Grace looked at the clock. It was two-thirty. She had an hour before her first lesson, giving her time to move all the papers and clutter out of sight and to make the visible portions of her home presentable. Some of the pressure for clean-house perfection was lifted since Maureen wouldn't be coming with Natalie. Even while delivering her rapid fire monologues, Maureen had an amazing talent for scanning the house, eyes darting all over as if she were some sort of human high tech surveillance machine searching for signs of dust or poor decorating taste. As Grace tidied the house, she found herself thinking about meeting Brian's son later at Natalie's lesson and wondered how he might have coped with his parents' divorce and his father's new family. She remembered the life altering challenges her parents' divorce created for her and then, the thing she swore as a young girl she would never do if she were to marry and have children, her own divorce. Although she had come to understand that impermanence is a fact of life and that it is naively optimistic to believe anything should be an exception, she still regretted the pain divorce had brought to her sons' lives. There was no way to avoid its impact on them, but she did everything in her power to minimize its damage. Only time would tell if she succeeded.

The fire was stoked, a pot of tea steeping, and candles were lit to warm the dim afternoon light that would soon fade to darkness. As she lit each candle, Grace silently brought to mind the students she would be teaching and her intention to be present for whatever they would need most. This helped her segue from the earlier preoccupations of her day into teaching.

Grace had told all her students that her front door would be unlocked and that they should let themselves in. If someone was still having their lesson when they arrived, they waited downstairs in the room with the old couches that were so well worn that they sank to embrace whoever sat in them. This was the same room that held the wood stove and whose warmth was an immediate comfort from the biting cold outside. For the older students, there was a cup of hot tea.

⌒

If even the thought to relieve
Living creatures of merely a headache
Is a beneficial intention
Endowed with infinite goodness,

Then what need is there to mention
The wish to dispel their inconceivable misery,
Wishing every single one of them,
To realize boundless good qualities?
I. v. 21, 22

How Generosity Works

Three students had come and gone before a timid knock interrupted the fourth. Even with a let-yourself-in policy, there were some who doubted its etiquette. Grace practically tiptoed to open the door while Jared kept playing. She smiled a silent "hello" and motioned for Natalie and her half brother to take a seat downstairs and returned quickly to her chair next to the piano bench until Jared's lesson was finished. They reviewed his practice instructions for the week before Grace walked with him to the door and then downstairs where Natalie was waiting.

"Hi, Natalie, this must be your brother." She walked towards the couch where they were sitting. "Hi, I'm Grace."

Natalie's brother fumbled to close the magazine he'd been looking through and stood to shake Grace's extended hand.

"Hey, I'm Troy."

"Maureen said you'd be waiting here while Natalie has her lesson. Would you like a cup of tea?"

"Uh, sure. Okay."

"Herbal? Regular?"

"Anything's good."

"Cream, sugar, honey, or lemon?"

"Um, honey and lemon please."

She poured the tea into a heavy mug, floated a slice of lemon, and stirred in three generous globs of honey before placing it on the table next to Troy. The steam lifted from the mug in multiple spirals under the reading lamp, and with it, the scent of black tea soaked in lemon.

"Natalie, I'll be right with you. Go ahead and get your music ready and warm up with scales."

Grace loaded two more logs into the stove. She adjusted their placement with the poker to keep them from smothering the burning logs beneath them before latching the stove door shut. One of these days, she noted to herself, she had to figure out how to oil the squeak out of that latch.

On her way out of the room to join Natalie, she turned to Troy who seemed not quite sure what to do with himself. "Make yourself at home—you're welcome to look through the bookshelf if you get bored with the magazines."

"Okay. Thanks."

Natalie was onto the D Major scale by the time Grace sat down. Hands together, she inched her way up the keyboard, hesitating just a little before finding C#, and then on up to D.

"Let's try that again," Grace said. "The second and third time always brings more confidence."

Grace could tell that Natalie's home practice was inconsistent. But she also understood that her mother loaded her with activities. Dance lessons, school play rehearsals, gymnastics, and a social schedule were crowded into a busy week. So, Natalie's lessons flowed between instruction, practice, and a lot of space to simply enjoy the feeling of playing music.

"Good, Natalie," Grace said. "How's the sonatina?"

Natalie opened her book to the sonatina and put her hands on the keys.

"Before you begin, Natalie, look at the first few measures and hear the notes in your mind; hear the music the way you want it to sound."

Everything begins with a thought. Grace knew that life flows more harmoniously when the outcome we want can be vividly pictured in our imagination or—in the case of playing a piece of music—by vividly hearing it in the mind. Then, the mechanics and logistics become clearer, and the steps taken in that direction more deliberate. This was effective for playing a piece of music and was also a way for Grace's students to sample a taste of what Buddhists call mindfulness.

Natalie had taken every instruction very seriously. With Troy downstairs, and hoping to impress him, she was determined to do her best. She looked at the music, her eyes following it note-by-note. She did exactly what Grace had said to do and was *really* trying to hear the music in her mind.

"Okay. Take it at a slow tempo, and with a steady beat." Grace counted four beats, "1, 2, 3, and 4, and . . . " Natalie began to play without interrupting her focus. Even though it went slowly, her playing flowed with only a few rough spots until she reached the end of the sonatina.

Natalie asked, "Can I play 'Joy to the World' for Troy?"

Christmas was already three weeks in the past, but it takes awhile for kids to let go of Christmas. "Of course," Grace said. "Go get him."

Natalie spun around and off the piano bench to get Troy.

Outside, Grace could hear the heavy grinding and clanking of sand trucks barreling down the road. She looked out the window and, in the light of the streetlamp, saw that snow had begun to fall. She could tell by the density of the snowflakes that this was going to be much more than a dusting.

Troy followed Natalie into the room carrying a book with his index finger stuck between its pages to hold his place. Elbow-height to Troy, Natalie pulled him by the arm to sit in the green chair by the window. When he sat down and held the book in his lap, the Buddha sitting in the Zen garden was gazing directly at Grace. Recalling the launching pad this book had been for her, seeing it now with Troy was one of those intersecting moments some call chance but Grace understood as karmic. Time stood still as it often will when something that feels like a *deja vu* inserts itself into a split second. The snow was the only thing that continued to move, like specks of glass in a spotlight, while the *deja vu* registered and then released but not without leaving its mark.

After she had positioned her brother where she wanted him, Natalie circled back to the piano and slid onto the bench. Rarely had Grace seen Natalie this animated. Judging by the expression on Troy's face, this was a new side of Natalie for him as well. Like someone who has just been given an award for something he didn't realize he had done, there was an amused humility that lit his face—forming the first smile that Troy had offered anyone for days.

Grace whispered a reminder to Natalie, "Hear it in your mind first . . . "

Natalie placed her hands on the keys, paused, and then played with more strength than one might expect from small hands. Careful not to lose his place in the book, Troy opened it to rest page-side down on the table next to him so his hands were free to applaud. Grace watched their eyes meet, felt the reverberation of the *deja vu* of a few minutes earlier, and drew in a slow, deep breath to center and absorb the moment. The Buddha on the book cover appeared to be doing the same.

"You guys better get home before the roads get icy. Natalie, if you're lucky, maybe you'll have a snow day off from school tomorrow." On a night that shows promise of snow, most kids offer some form of prayer asking for a mountain of snow to close the schools.

Grace watched Troy read something on the page he had the book opened to while Natalie gathered her music into her bookbag. "Troy, if you're interested in reading that book, you can take it home with you."

How Generosity Works

"Really? Thank you. I took a class in Asian Studies when I was in school. It was one of the only classes I actually learned something in . . . " He almost said more, but let his voice drop like you do when you realize the story you're about to tell is more involved than you have either time or energy to tell.

Grace understood. Sensing his sadness, she didn't pry. She offered the first thought that came to her mind. "The things we learn don't always make their way onto a college transcript, but many times they wind up being the more crucial things because they help us find our way in life." And then, to fill the silence that was almost awkward in its potency, she added, "I hope you'll enjoy that book . . . it has a way of finding people at just the right time."

They said their goodbyes in the hallway. Natalie and Troy put on their boots, coats, hats, and gloves and fluffed their way through the snow down the driveway. Grace watched them drive around the bend; the back end of their truck skidded and tugged a little to the right before making it all the way up the hill.

Thus by the virtue collected
Through all that I have done,
May the pain of every living creature
Be completely cleared away.

May I be the doctor, the medicine
And may I be the nurse
For all sick beings in the world,
Until everyone is healed.
III. v. 7, 8

The snow was falling fast, and Grace needed to restock the supply of firewood she kept inside before it got too wet from the snow. Bundling up in the heavy parka her sons had outgrown, fur lined boots that zipped over her jeans, thick gloves, a scarf, and a wool hat, she headed out to the woodpile. A faded red plastic toboggan that she pulled by a rope slid along behind her. One log at a time, she loaded the wood into the toboggan, filling it only as full as she could without logs spilling out on the return trip to the house. It took a few armloads to empty the toboggan—knocking the snow off her boots each time she entered the house to stack the wood against the wall near the wood stove. She enjoyed the moistness of the snow melting on her cheeks while she repeated the trip to the woodpile a few more times.

The night sky in a heavy snow is lit differently than on other nights. Depending on the phase of the moon, you might see a slight rainbow circling its hazy glow, like a lighthouse in a foggy sea. There is an unmistakable feeling of coziness, or maybe even love, that fills the air when it blends with wood smoke. Not ready to close herself back into her house, she walked down the narrow road that led to the edge of the woods. Grace had a small world to herself where footsteps make no sound and night transforms into a timeless and silent landscape in which falling ice crystals take the place of stars.

A gust of wind blew, and Grace adjusted her scarf a little more snugly to keep the snow and wind from blowing down her neck and under her jacket. She was still thinking about Troy. He was probably only a few years younger than her sons and since her mothering gene was perennially active, her concern extended easily to others. Another strong gust of wind sent the snow swirling, stinging her face like a moving cloud of tiny needles, and Grace turned her back to the wind until it settled. By the time she wound her way back to her house, the toboggan tracks and her earlier footsteps were barely noticeable indentations in the blanket of snow.

She took off her wet boots and clothes and spread them out to dry on the stone hearth. As she was draping her coat over a chair, the image of Troy's truck struggling to climb the hill came to mind. The traffic from people returning home from work keeps enough heat on the main roads to make driving okay, but people can get stuck on the back roads if they're not plowed and sanded. She thought about calling the Reilly's house to make sure Troy and Natalie arrived safely, but she would have expected Maureen to call if they hadn't made it back home. Even so, she wanted concrete reassurance so she could put the concern to rest and picked up the phone to call.

An impatient voice answered the phone. "Hello?"

"Hi, Maureen, it's Grace." That voice was so frantic she wanted to get to the point quickly. "The roads are pretty dicey out there, and I just wanted to make sure that Natalie and Troy made it home okay."

"Yeah, they got home about half an hour ago." Then, a burdened sigh, "With this snow, everyone will be home tomorrow." That weight-of-the-world martyr voice was speaking again. Grace reminded herself to be patient. "Having Troy here is just too much. I can't stand it. Brian's ex-wife sold her house and moved into a small apartment, so he can't stay with her. Now we're stuck with him, and I'm already at the end of my rope. I told Brian he's got to get him back into another school for next semester. It doesn't even feel like my house anymore with him here. Just the sight of him drives me up a wall."

Grace could barely believe what she was hearing. In that moment, the pieces came together like metal filings under a magnet—the *deja vu*, the book, the conversation before Troy left. She couldn't have been more grateful for call waiting when Maureen announced that she had another call coming through. They quickly said goodbye, and Grace stood there with the phone in her hand, staring out the window but seeing nothing. Her mind was somewhere else.

May I be a protector for those without one,
A guide for all travelers on the way;
May I be a bridge, a boat and a ship
For all who wish to cross (the water).

May I be an island for those who seek one,
And a lamp for those desiring light,
May I be a bed for all who wish to rest
And a servant for all who want a servant.

May I be a wishing jewel, a magic vase,
Powerful mantras and great medicine,
May I become a wish-fulfilling tree
And a cow of plenty for the world.
III. v. 18, 19, 20

The following week brought a January thaw. Icicles and clumps of snow dropped from the roofs, and melting snowbanks carved miniature streams into the sand on the roads. Water was trickling through gutters and splashing into the drain grates on the streets. People scraped snow shovels to clear their driveways of the softening patches of snow and slush before they could freeze to ice when the sun went down. Neighbors greeted each other from their driveways. Conversation about the weather is a favorite topic in New England— there is always something new and different on the horizon, and people love to discuss the predictions for what is coming next. When they have the inside scoop from television news, they speak as if they have visited the oracle and carry the voice of authority to prove it. Grace didn't have a television but the weather revealed itself to her by the smells in the air, the rainbow rings around the moon, or by how tightly the rhododendron leaves curled. Nature, she thought, was the perfect working model to demonstrate the ever-changing essence of life, its interdependence in order to exist as it does, and the physics of cause and effect, or karma.

From beyond the droning sound of snow shovels scraping asphalt, Grace heard a lilting melody of reggae music. It grew louder as an old blue pickup truck came around the bend and pulled to stop at the end of Grace's driveway. When he rolled his window down, Grace realized it was Troy.

"Hey, Grace! I was just up the road at my friend's house. I saw you," he turned the music off, "and I wanted to thank you for what you said the other day— about there being important things to learn that aren't always taught in college."

Snow shovel in hand, Grace walked closer to Troy's truck. "Oh? Well, I'm glad if it helped."

"Yeah, it really did help—kinda like getting a different perspective on all that's gone down."

"Well, I gather it's been a tough year for you. Was this your first semester away at school?" Grace was aware of the delicate balance between giving someone space to speak freely and not being intrusive. The coldness of what Maureen had said about Troy was disturbing and triggered a strong urge to offer anything that might help him find his way.

"No," he answered, "but there've been a lot of changes, and I guess that I'm just questioning a lot."

"Well," she said, "that means your mind is working and that's a good thing . . . Are you in a hurry? Would you like to come in for some tea?"

He looked at the clock on the dashboard of his truck. "Yeah, okay. I've got time. Thanks." Troy pulled his truck into the driveway to park and followed Grace into the house.

    ⌒

May I become an inexhaustible treasure
For those who are poor and destitute;
May I turn into all things they could need
And be placed close beside them.
III. v. 10

Maybe it was the warmth of the wood stove and the different sort of heat it fills a home with, or the way sunlight poured through the windows that made Troy feel as if he'd entered a different realm. Whatever it was, it carried a feeling of home, and with it, the recognition that it had been years since he had one.

Grace filled the teakettle with water and took some mugs out of the cupboard. Like the unmetered pause before a new movement in a piece of music, she let silence clear its space so a new dynamic could settle into the room.

It was Troy who broke the silence. "So, I've been reading your book about Buddhism, and I'm trying to understand the karma thing and why everything I do seems to turn out wrong."

Grace stood at the kitchen counter, squeezing the water from the teabags by nesting them in a spoon and wrapping the attached string around itself several times. She watched the last drips of tea-darkened water leave the teabag as her mind was searching for the best way to respond. She balanced the teabag on the spoon while she considered what Troy was asking, and then placed it on the small china saucer. "Well, those are almost two different questions, so maybe I'll try to answer the part about karma first."

She cut two thin slices of lemon and put one in each of the mugs. Straining to open the honey jar she explained, "Karma works like seeds. For example, what will grow if you plant an apple seed?"

"An apple tree."

She turned on the faucet to rinse the honey and lemon juice off her hands and dried them on the dishtowel that was hanging on the cupboard door. "But then, what would happen if you planted an apple seed in the desert?"

"Not much. At least, not without a lot of help."

She poured an extra spoonful of honey in Troy's tea and stirred it slowly to let the honey dissolve. "So, in order for an apple tree to grow, it needs first a seed, then to be planted, and then it needs to have the right conditions like good soil, water, and sunlight, right?"

"Right," he answered.

Carrying a mug in each hand, she placed his on the table in front of him, and then her own across from him as she slid the wooden chair along the old oak floor and sat down. "So, thinking about karma as something like seeds, now consider the things people do, say, and think as all being seeds they plant in their lives."

Troy frowned. "How are the thoughts people think like seeds? They don't get planted anywhere."

"Well, if you think about it, the things you think about produce different feelings, right? If you think about something upsetting—like, if someone ever betrayed or hurt you—even if it happened a long time ago, it can still have an effect on you. Your body might feel tense, and you might feel angry or sad. So, right then and there, the thought—or the seed—begins to take root."

"Okay, but—so what?—I mean, it's not like it's *doing* anything."

"Maybe it doesn't appear that way. But thoughts have varying intensity—a strong one, for instance, will have more powerful results—the results can either be things we consider to be good, or things we consider to be bad. I think you might even be able to think about how you feel as being the quality indicator of the karmic result of your thought."

Grace knew there was always a simple way to explain complex things, but sometimes it could take awhile to find the right method depending on who she was talking to. "So, let me try to come up with an example. It could be that for some reason, something reminds you of a time when you were in high school and saw some guy giving one of your friends a hard time—maybe it got physical, and he knocked your friend over. Just *thinking* about it you remember your outrage and how you went running after the guy, but he had a group of his friends with him, and you knew you were outnumbered and couldn't do what you wanted to do." Grace stopped for a moment to gather her thoughts, which included wondering how and why she came up with that scenario. It was too late to do anything except to keep working with it, so she continued. "Just by remembering this, your body begins to feel tense, you recall your anger—you actually *feel* your anger, and, already, your *mind* has been changed by these thoughts—you're not a happy camper at this moment, are you?"

"No, not at all." Troy actually laughed.

"So, already that little karmic seed has begun to spread its roots and sprout some leaves, right?"

"Okay . . . I guess so," he said.

"But, what if at the time when you're remembering this incident, you happen to be driving and another driver—for this story, let's make it be a guy around your age—enters an intersection without stopping and nearly hits your car. You have to quickly swerve out of the way. Now you're *really* mad, and you slam on your horn and yell a string of words out the window that wouldn't be polite for me to repeat," she smiled at Troy, "and before you know it, your heart's pounding, and you're driving after the guy still screaming at him until you manage to pull up alongside him at the next stoplight." Again, she wondered if this illustration was actually going to help, but she was on a roll with it, and Troy seemed to be drawn into the story with her. "At this point, several possibilities exist, right? The other driver might be getting mad too and start yelling and swearing at you and calling you out, so you explode with rage, jump out of your car, and he gets out of his car, and then all hell breaks loose. Do you see how the seed just starts to grow wild, like a weed on steroids?"

Troy agreed and laughed a little, but it wasn't an amused laugh so much as one that revealed this was a scene he could easily imagine.

"Another possibility is the other driver might have the wherewithal and composure to roll down his window and say, 'I'm *really* sorry, man—I made a really bad move, and I'm glad you were able to get out of the way. I hope you're okay.'" She waited for that potentiality to soak in. "What karmic seed did he just plant, and what happens to that out of control weed on steroids?"

"Well, I'd like to think that I wouldn't get out of my car and go after him. I'd probably feel a little embarrassed, and I don't know if I would suddenly stop being pissed off, but later in the day—whether or not I'd admit it to anyone—I'd be glad that I didn't get into a fight."

He hadn't answered the first part of her question, so she asked him again, "But what karmic seed did the other guy plant?"

"A nice one?"

Maybe she was being too obtuse. "Yes—definitely a nice one. It worked a little like a harmless weed-killer, didn't it? The other driver planted the karmic seed of kindness. And, if you spend some time thinking about it, you might see how kindness has more power than anger."

She sipped her tea and tried not to be too obvious as she watched his face for signs of some sort of recognition and understanding. He was playing with the lemon in his tea, absently making it turn circles inside the cup.

She continued, "Does that help you to understand karma—and how our thoughts, actions, and speech are all both the causes and the results, or karma, for things that happen in our lives?"

"Yeah, actually it does help. Thanks." He wiped his wet fingers on his jeans.

"Good," she said. "So, do you want to go on to the second part of your question? The part about why it feels as if the things you do don't turn out well? Or is that enough to think about for one day?"

"Actually, yeah—go for it!" He looked at Grace and smiled.

"Okay." With her elbows resting on the table, she held her tea in both hands and blew across the top to cool it before she took a sip. "The Buddhists speak in terms of countless lifetimes, and that the lives we are living now are the karmic results of lives we've lived before. And then, our future lives will be the karmic result of the cumulative lives we've lived, including this one now. But, for some people, that's a tall order to get their minds around. Even if considering past or future lives seems too out there, we can still benefit by considering karma as it applies only to this present life."

Troy shifted around in his chair and drummed his hands on his thighs, "Yeah, I think I'm a little more comfortable just sticking to this lifetime—it's the only one I know about, even though I feel a little clueless about what I'm doing with it."

"Okay." Grace leaned forward. "So, remember how our actions—whether in the form of thought, speech, or some sort of physical action—are like seeds we plant?"

"Yeah." He was swirling the lemon around in his tea again.

Grace asked, "What determines whether or not the seed we plant is going to grow into something like an out-of-control weed that is destructive, or a beautiful flower or fruit-bearing plant like an apple tree?"

Troy answered without hesitating, "Well, based on the story you used as an example, I'd say it has to do with your state of mind when you're doing whatever it is you're doing."

Grace agreed and went on. "There are actions that are destructive and others that bring about good things, right? And when we think a little further, we realize that underneath every action is some sort of motivation. Sometimes that motivation can be a little clouded—even to ourselves. In other words, sometimes

How Generosity Works

we zip around in life doing things in some sort of reflexive way, and we don't even question *why* we're doing whatever it is we're doing." Grace was aware that she was struggling to keep things simple and wasn't convinced that she was succeeding.

Troy tilted his head, his eyes searching the corner of the ceiling. Not in the way Maureen would have been looking for cobwebs or noting that the walls were in dire need of paint. But more in the way it would be if it were possible to see through the walls into the landscape on the other side.

She watched him piece things together and then continued. "Simply put, there are destructive actions, and there are negative motivations that can make them even more destructive. The flip side is that there are good actions or what the Buddhists call virtuous actions. Virtuous actions bring about positive results. And, since we're talking about seeds and apple trees, we could say that virtuous motivations become the fertilizer that will produce the best quality fruit. Essentially, everything we do is a process of planting seeds that will produce our future karma." The darkening sky, laced with crimson streaks, brought afternoon shadows that lowered themselves across the room. Grace reached to turn on the brass lamp that sat on the table. "So, if things seem to have not gone well for you, it doesn't mean you are a bad person doomed to live a karmic nightmare. Instead, if you reflect on things you have done and what your actual motivations may have been, you will begin to see where a different understanding could have produced different actions and then, a different result." Her eyes met his, and in the lamplight she could see his eyes moistening. "It also means you have an opportunity to reevaluate what you would like your future to include and practice planting the appropriate seeds and providing them with the right conditions so the fruit they produce is sweet!"

Just as a flash of lightning on a dark, cloudy night
For an instant brightly illuminates all,
Likewise in this world, through the might of the Buddha,
A wholesome thought rarely and briefly appears.

Hence virtue is perpetually feeble,
The great strength of immorality being extremely intense,
And except for a Fully Awakened Mind,
By what other virtue will it be overcome?
I. v. 5, 6

Neither Grace nor Troy spoke while the traces of their conversation filled the room and floated around each of them like a long silk scarf that carried an enchanted spell. The silence was a fermata, held until the tones blended and dissolved into silence. The sounds in the room reintroduced themselves as if they too had been silent, and the ticking clock brought Troy's attention to the time. "Uh oh. I'm supposed to pick Natalie up from her friend's house and get her home for dinner. Maureen's gonna freak out if I'm late."

Grace laughed and slid her chair out from the table to stand. "She runs a pretty tight ship, so you better get going." They walked together to the door where Troy put his boots on. Grace caught herself holding his coat in her reflexive motherly mode and immediately reminded herself to simply hand it to him. Troy looked at the piano on the old, threadbare Persian rug and said, "If Maureen let's me, I'll bring Natalie to her lesson again this week."

Grace said, "I'm sure if you offer, she'll appreciate your help and won't turn you down."

With more cynicism than optimism in his voice he said, "Yeah, maybe." He zipped up his coat and dug his keys from the pocket. "Thanks for the tea and for the conversation. There's so much to think about;

I think it'll help me weigh out some decisions I have to make."

"You're very welcome. I enjoyed the visit, and I'll hope to see you in a few days." Grace turned the porch light on and watched Troy jog to his truck. She closed the door and walked downstairs to stoke the fire.

Just like space
And the great elements such as earth,
May I always support the lives
of all the boundless creatures.

And until they pass away from pain,
May I also be the source of life
For all the realms of varied beings
That reach unto the ends of space.
III. v. 21, 22

Pulling the curtains closed over the windows, her eyes rested on a photograph taken of her sons when they were four and six years old. Two little boys dressed in miniature army uniforms and helmets, smiling across time through the picture frame. The sensation of missing them rose and struck like a rogue wave. She missed their younger antics, Nathan's rambunctious sense of humor and playful energy that never stopped and Miles's sweet and tender ways that would carry a fistful of wild flowers home after a weekend with their father. She missed the exuberance that charged through the house—and how their two bodies could stampede with the force of twenty.

Memories have a way of getting caught in the crossfire between past and present where decades disappear in a mind that holds onto things colored by either love or pain. Any memory—good or bad—can spring to life and hold the mind captive to longing or hatred. Grace hadn't yet achieved mastery over these things, but she had learned to recognize them when they showed up. She knew that life is an ever-flowing fountain of change, and holding onto things in an attached way is like trying to squeeze a stream of water as if you could hold it still in your hand. Not only is it impossible, but the pressure in the tightened fist will eventually bring pain. Releasing the grip is where freedom exists to truly enjoy what is, what has been, and what is yet to be.

She also understood that it was one thing to know these things and quite another to live by them.

Releasing the grip, no matter how promising, has the intimidating sensation of destroying the emotional ground you stand on. It takes intellectual understanding combined with actual practice to even begin to soften the grip. Grace was accustomed to hours upon hours of practice to learn difficult pieces on the piano. Until she was able to master the hand's choreography within a phrase, demanding passages were clumsy. By isolating the phrase and practicing it over and over again, the notes eventually poured from her fingers like water over glass. The practice of mindfulness works in a similar way by slowing things down to feel the pulse of what is really going on and then taking it apart—note by note—distilling it down to its truth.

Whenever a negative emotion creeps in, there is clinging or grasping at its root. In truth, it is not to the object or the person that we are clinging, but it is to *ourselves* we cling as if we require that special object or that special person to sustain our existence. Buddhists call this condition self-grasping, and they would also add that as the root cause, it is responsible for unhappiness. Clinging to a person—or to the memory of them—as if they are the sustainer of life and happiness is not only inaccurate, but through clinging, love is tainted with conditionality. In other words, the other person's existence is being viewed as if it is for one's own happiness. By gently opening the clenched fist, the hand is open to experience a pure love, a love that is motivated by a deep desire for the happiness of others. It wasn't that Grace needed to stop loving her sons, or to not enjoy the warm memories shared with them. She knew she simply needed to release her grip, smile in gratitude for the memory, and allow love to flow without grasping or conditions.

Slipping into a pair of boots and wrapping an old paisley down comforter around herself, Grace walked outside to her back patio, a nightly ritual that began when Paul left their home and marriage. In previous years, after she read to the boys and tucked them in for the night, it was the night sky that answered her when she said "good night." Although there were chairs on the patio that she could sit in, she mostly preferred to stand. The constellations passed overhead as the seasons carried Orion, Scorpio, and Cassiopeia across the sky. It didn't matter if it was overcast, in her solitude she was comforted by their presence. Grace was growing older under the watchful eye of the traveling constellations. She looked up, as she often did, first to find the moon and then to see what constellation she might recognize in the sky. Clouds had moved into the night and no stars could be seen, but the lights from town infused the sky with a soft glow. The sensation of cold moisture in the air and the familiar ring around the moon foretold that snow was on its way.

⌐⌐

Grace opened her eyes to a snow globe world the next morning. The hypnotic effect of watching snowflakes from under a bundle of blankets can easily send you back into sleep, pursuing threads of dreams that want to know their endings. Having drifted back to sleep under the weight of cozy blankets and heavy eyes, Grace was startled awake by the sound of plows thundering down the road, ferociously grinding against the pavement. Preparing herself for the cold room she was about to confront, in one fluid motion she pulled the blankets off, rolled upright and out of bed.

She had slept so late that only a few embers remained in the thick pile of ashes that covered the bottom of the stove. She scooped the ashes into a cast iron bucket, tossed several sheets of crumpled newspaper into the stove that she covered with kindling, and lit a match to get the fire started again. The house was cold, and it would take awhile to heat. Even with its late start, the morning routine was underway, and meditation was not to be bypassed. Sitting on her cushion, Grace brought her attention to her breath and mentally followed its passage through inhaling and exhaling. Rinpoche had taught her, on each exhale, to visualize a beautiful, fresh flower in her lower abdomen. It didn't matter what type of flower, and while it was okay if the flower changed with each exhale, the important thing was that the image of the flower be fresh. Since her mind had jumpstarted with the realization that she had overslept, she was already distracted by things she wanted to do before the snow piled up. This particular meditation offered something simple to focus her attention on and would bring her mind back to its calm state. We can't always control the circumstances we encounter, but we can control how we greet them. Meditation never failed to clear the static of agitation and pave the way for a more peaceful day.

⌣

Those who wish to destroy the many sorrows of their
conditioned existence,
Those who wish all beings to experience a multitude
of joys,
And those who wish to experience much happiness
Should never forsake the Awakening Mind.

I. v. 8

Grace poured her coffee and carried it, sipping as she washed her face and got dressed. There was a chance she would be snowed in for a day or two, and she needed groceries—most importantly, she needed coffee and cream. Racing against the falling snow, practicality reigned over glamour, and Grace left her house bundled in layers that added a lumpy roundness under her coat. She caught a glimpse of herself in the mirror as she walked toward the door and reminded herself, "All appearances are just a mental projection, so just get over it." She swept the snow off her car and started the engine to defrost the windows while she shoveled a path out of her driveway.

Grace wasn't the only one scrambling to get groceries. The store owner looked busy but happy with a shop full of customers and money pouring in almost as fast as the snow fell. Determined to get in and out of the store quickly, Grace weaved her way between people and shopping carts. As she turned down the last aisle heading for the cash register, Maureen walked toward her with a basket already filled to capacity.

"Hi, Grace." Immediately, the sighing began, "Oh my God, I'm so fed up with this weather. We're getting a foot of snow." Maureen looked beyond Grace as if she needed to see who else was in the store. "I told Brian he's taking Natalie and me to Florida for spring break in February." Maureen's eyes scoured Grace's ensemble with no attempt to be discreet.

"Really? We're getting a foot?" Grace asked, pretending not to notice her outfit was being scrutinized.

"Yeah. That's what I heard this morning." Maureen took a box of brownie mix off the shelf and put it in her basket.

Grace felt anger rising up within her as she recalled Maureen's vicious complaints about Troy. She also remembered that karma was always ripening and that nothing good would come in the presence of anger. Rinpoche taught that anger, greed, and delusion are states of mind that arise from ignorance of our true nature, which is the awakened heart of wisdom and compassion. Maureen's unpleasant behaviors were classic manifestations of someone suffering from ignorance. Remembering this released a flood of compassion that poured through Grace's body with a force that took her by surprise. She observed Maureen's unhappiness and that her way of commanding people in her life was a desperate attempt to make her world more stable. The same strong desire that moved Grace to help all those she loved and cared about spilled over into a strong wish to help Maureen.

"I'm glad I ran into you because I wanted to tell you how well Natalie played at her lesson last week. She even gave a recital for Troy." As soon as she mentioned Troy's name, she worried that she might have made a mistake. "I know blending families can be difficult, so it was good to see how nicely they are getting along."

"Yeah, it's not easy. At least Brian's other kids are older and live on their own. I'm counting the days until Troy gets out of the house." She picked up a box of cake mix and was speedreading the directions before she tossed it into her cart. "But he doesn't have any place to go yet, and Brian won't make him stay with his mother. With the amount of money Brian has to send her every month, she could have rented a bigger apartment."

Grace didn't want to touch that comment, so she shifted the conversation away from Brian, money, and the ex-wife. "Last time we talked, you said you wanted him to get into another school. Is that what Troy wants as well?"

"Oh," she groaned, "he doesn't know what the hell he wants." As she talked, she inspected her manicure, and then rocked her left hand slightly to watch the light sparkle in her diamond. "He screwed up so badly that he has to take this semester off. Now he is taking night classes at the community college, and he can try again next semester."

"Well, if it's of any comfort, it took me awhile before I did well as a student. It wasn't until I studied music that I developed the discipline and desire to do well." She smiled at Maureen. "Don't worry, he won't live with you forever. I'm sure he's as eager to be on his own as you are to have him out. In the meantime, at least you have someone available to help drive Natalie places."

Maureen laughed, "Well, if he's eager to do anything, it's a mystery to me." Now she was busy plucking lint off her jacket. "All he does is close himself into his room and either read some stupid book about God-knows-what or play his guitar."

"Well, there are certainly worse things young guys can get themselves wrapped up in." Grace looked out the store's front window. "Maureen, look at that snow. We better get going or we'll be setting up camp in this store."

"Okay. Bye." Maureen and her cart were quickly in motion. She spoke loudly as she walked away, "I won't see you this week. I'm gonna have Troy take Natalie to her lesson on Thursday."

Grace said "goodbye" even though Maureen couldn't hear her. Continuing to the checkout line, she mentally repeated over and over again, "May Maureen be happy and at peace, and may her heart be filled with joy."

By the time Grace arrived back home, the snow had piled perfectly balanced, leveled cushions of white that covered each limb and twig of every tree, porch railing, phone line, and parked car with infallible precision, leaving no exposed spot of landscape uncovered. The day continued on under the mystical spell that snowstorms carry within their heavy clouds bringing only a vague sense of time's passing, while snow fell silently onto the fields. Stone walls shape-shifted into long rows of featherbeds, and the pond, thick with ice beneath the snow, into a shallow crater in the silvery landscape. The hedges and bare-branched forsythia that bordered the garden lowered themselves under the weight of the snow, and the last snowflakes fell as dusk ushered in the night, putting the finishing touches on the work of a silent sculptor.

~

Likewise for the sake of all that lives
Do I give birth to an Awakening Mind,
And likewise shall I, too,
Successively follow the practices.
III. v. 24

On Thursday morning, sunlight bounced between the sky and the snow-covered earth, like a massive mirror telegraphing messages between the spheres. Grace spent the morning at the piano, practicing some new pieces and refreshing others she hadn't touched for months. She reserved her favorite, Chopin's *Nocturne in E Minor*, to play last. For Grace, this piece of music practically played itself even though it was her own fingers that found the keys and her own body that leaned into its phrases. Playing this music had the power to bring the scattered fragments of a broken heart together—even if only temporarily. According to Buddhists, the lasting method for healing a broken heart is to offer love and compassion to others, and Grace was practicing this as well.

Later that afternoon when Troy opened the front door to bring Natalie for her lesson, Grace noticed an unusual light in his eyes. As with the green flash at sunset, it lasted for only an instant. Could it have been the flash of the awakened mind of bodhicitta— the awakened heart and mind that carries the powerful wish for all beings to be free of suffering? Whatever it was, Grace felt the causes and conditions that brought him into her home, that drew him to that particular book, and that raised the questions he sought answers to were all things that needed to be paid attention to. Within that instant, Grace sealed her conviction that helping Troy move beyond the unhappy crossroads where he stood was not only something she wanted to do, but it was something she was compelled to do. Even though her attention turned to working with Natalie, the energy of her determination had a momentum that was already in motion.

When Natalie's lesson was finished, Troy walked over to the piano and sat next to her on the piano bench. "Ready, Nat?" She didn't answer, but she smiled and positioned her two index fingers on F and G and waited for her entrance while Troy began to bang out the bass part of "Chopsticks." After several repetitions, Troy slowed the tempo, and Natalie followed his cue to end.

"Fabulous!" Grace applauded. "'Chopsticks' is one of my favorite pieces of music. I couldn't think of a better finale to my day. Thank you."

Troy wrapped his arm around Natalie and squeezed her against his side. She smiled and wriggled off the bench and reached to hug Grace. With her arms around Natalie, Grace spoke to Troy from behind Natalie's shoulder, "I knew you played the guitar, but I didn't know you played the piano too." She patted Natalie on the back, completing the hug. Natalie twirled ballerina circles in the center of the room while Grace and Troy talked.

"Well, I wouldn't exactly call it playing the piano, but yeah, I noodle around a bit. How'd you know I play the guitar?" Troy drummed his hands against his thighs to a rhythm that must have been a constant sound track in his own mind.

"The other day before the snowstorm, I ran into Maureen at the grocery store, and she mentioned that you've been playing the guitar a lot since you've been home." Grace hoped her tone of voice concealed the negativity that had come from Maureen.

"She thinks it's a waste of time, so I'm surprised she even bothered mentioning it." Troy's drumming had stopped. He studied the keys on the keyboard and absentmindedly plunked out a scale.

"Mommy's just grouchy, Troy." Natalie came back toward the piano bench and leaned with both hands on the bench and looked up to see Troy's face. "She doesn't really think you're wasting time, she just complains a lot." She moved away from the bench again, practicing another ballet position, "Anyway, I love when you play the guitar."

"Thanks, Nat." Troy glanced at the bookshelves in the room and then spoke to Grace again, "I'm still reading that book you gave me. I like it a lot. But I'm not a real fast reader, so I hope you don't mind that I've still got it."

Grace leaned forward, her folded arms resting on her lap. "Troy, I gave you that book as a gift. I'm really glad you're enjoying reading it." She sat back in her chair again and stretched, clasping her hands behind her head. "Besides, I can always find another copy if I want one." Picking up her interest in knowing more about Troy's music, she shifted the subject back again. "Troy, have you taken lessons, or did you teach yourself how to play the guitar?"

Spreading both hands over the keys, Troy began playing octaves slowly up the keyboard. "I had some lessons on the guitar when I was younger and remember some things from music class in school, but mostly I've just figured things out myself."

"I can teach you some music theory if you'd like," Grace said. "The piano works really well for helping to understand harmony and stuff like that because it's so easy to actually see how scales form and how intervals work on the keyboard." People can learn a lot on their own and with the help of books, but as Grace had learned through meeting Rinpoche, the rocket fuel for learning anything comes from having the right teacher. Grace waited before she said anything more—he might have been perfectly content with what he already knew. And if he was anything like her sons, free time was something to spend with friends, not with women older than their mothers.

"Seriously?" Troy stopped playing octaves, and his face softened into a smile. "I'd love to learn all that. I've thought about studying music in college, but there's no way I could without knowing how to read music. I know I'd need a stronger background."

"Well, let's change that." Grace stood up to look at her calendar. "I've got time on Tuesdays around three o'clock. How about you?"

"I can do that," he answered.

"Do you want to start this coming Tuesday?" Grace called out from the next room where she stood facing the calendar that hung on the wall.

"Yeah. Definitely. I work breakfast and lunch at the diner in town, so I'll come here right after work." He laughed, "I might smell like home fries and bacon though—hope you don't mind."

"No problem," Grace said as she came back into the room where Natalie was lying on the floor, tracing the designs on the rug with her fingers.

"C'mon, Nat." Troy reached over to tug on Natalie's braid. "Get your stuff together. I've gotta get you home for dinner."

Natalie whined, "But I hate fish. I don't wanna go."

Troy stood and bent to lift Natalie up to her feet. "Yeah, but we've gotta go."

She began to laugh and playfully threw herself back down onto the floor. "No! It smells disgusting. I don't want to go—Mommy's going to make me eat fish."

Troy picked her up again. "Just sneak your fish onto my plate when she's not looking. I'll eat it for you."

"Okay." Natalie ran to the door and put her boots and coat on while Troy carried her books. "But don't eat my mashed potatoes or dessert."

"I won't. Just get in the truck before your mom gets mad at me for being late." He turned to look at Grace, "Thanks, Grace—I'll see you Tuesday." He opened the door and held Natalie's hand as they walked down the driveway.

"Goodbye, Grace!" Natalie yelled before she climbed into Troy's truck.

"Goodbye. See you soon!" Grace called back.

The glass on the storm door fogged over when the indoor heat met the cold outside. Grace lifted the handle on the door to open it and walked onto the front porch. She stood in the cold with her arms crossed tightly over themselves for warmth. Under the lamplight by her front door, each breath sent puffs of mist like steam into the air. She stood there only long enough to watch an airplane carve its path into the evening sky. Its lights flashed between Venus and the tree line before it disappeared behind the darkened hills. Back inside, she shivered off the cold that followed her in and added more wood to the fire in the stove. She stood close to the stove with her hands outstretched over it to absorb the heat radiating from its surface while she thought about the lessons she would begin teaching Troy the following week.

⌒

Gladly do I rejoice
In the virtue that relieves the misery
Of all those in unfortunate states
And that gives happiness to the suffering.
III. v. 1

Along with her invitation to teach Troy about music, Grace felt a deeper responsibility to help him understand that when pain and challenges enter our lives they carry the ingredients for alchemy. When our thoughts are disturbed by negativity, or when others treat us badly, there are skillful practices to reframe the way we perceive these situations to generate an entirely different experience. Through the power of wisdom, our challenges and painful experiences can be seen as treasures that become our path to freedom. If Troy could understand the role of compassion to transform his relationship with Maureen, he would have a profound experience that would lead him to see the nature of interconnectedness, and how each of us is responsible for the world we live in.

Grace climbed the stairs, and instead of fixing something for dinner, she walked past the piano, stepped over the pile of music scattered on the floor, and then down the hall to the small study that she used for meditation. Before taking her seat on the cushion, she stood with her eyes closed and pressed her hands together in front of her chest to prepare for prostrations. With the bodhichitta motivation to benefit all beings, she raised her hands above her head and touched the base of her palms to the crown of her head, symbolizing her connection with the idea of the enlightened body. She then lowered her joined hands to touch her throat, connecting with enlightened speech, and then lowered them once more to touch her heart, connecting with enlightened mind. Then, separating her hands, she leaned forward until her hands were on the floor in front of her, bent her knees to crouch, and rocked forward to bring her knees onto the floor, and then in one smooth motion, continued forward to touch her forehead to the floor. With the five points of the body touching the floor, the five disturbing emotions of anger, attachment, ignorance, pride and jealousy are said to be purified. Symbolically, they leave the body and disappear into the earth. Pushing off the floor with her hands, she stood again with the palms of her hands pressed together in front of her chest and repeated the process a second and then a third time.

Grace sat on her cushion and with her eyes closed, imagined the Buddha dissolving into one very bright light in front of her. She began to watch her breath as if it could be seen on the screen of her mind like a ribbon of light that poured in with each inhale from the light in front of her. In this way, she watched it stream into her body like water coming in through the pipes in a house and then out again with each exhale. She counted eleven breaths like this before she began a special meditation called tonglen. Tonglen, a Tibetan word that translates as taking and giving, is a healing visualization that uses difficult circumstances we encounter in life as a method to replace negativity with compassion and wisdom. The healing is for oneself, one another, and for all sentient beings. Just like falling dominoes, the things that harm one individual will harm others, and the things that benefit one will benefit all. Tonglen uses compassion to equalize all beings—in other words, there are no good guys or bad guys according to this view.

She began the tonglen practice by thinking of Troy and the pain and sadness he was experiencing and then held the image of him in her mind, imagining all his sadness and pain leaving his body in the form of thick and heavy dark smoke. She watched it gather into a black cloud outside his body, and then, inhaling, she drew it all into herself, taking all his sadness and pain from him. On her exhale, she sent light pouring out through her body to Troy, filling his body with a clear light. She saw him radiant and at peace. The joy she experienced by seeing him free of pain obliterated her own self-grasping and the darkness she had just breathed in. Next, she moved on to Maureen in her meditation. She needed to sort through a process of thinking that allowed her to generate a powerful feeling of love and compassion for her. Applying the wisdom of equanimity and the wisdom that comes from comprehending impermanence, she reinforced her understanding that concepts like "enemy" and "friend" are only temporary. The ultimate wish is for all beings to be free of suffering, not only a chosen group. As long as even one being is suffering, there can be no peace. Through this practice, Grace was able to feel love and compassion for Maureen. She saw the pain and suffering that Maureen carried within her and imagined it all leaving her body as she had for Troy. She visualized it in front of her, collected into a ball of dark smoke, and drew it into herself with her next inhale. Breathing out, she sent light pouring outward to Maureen. She repeated this several times until she was able to imagine Maureen filled with clear light—happy and at peace. The joy that Grace felt by seeing Maureen happy and free destroyed all traces of darkness she had breathed in and replaced it with light.

⌒

The moment an Awakening Mind arises
In those fettered and weak in the jail of cyclic existence,
They will be named a 'Child of the Sugatas,'
And will be revered by both humans and gods of the
world.

It is like the supreme fold-making elixir,
For it transforms the unclean body we have taken

Into the priceless jewel of a Buddha-Form.
Therefore firmly seize this Awakening Mind
I. v. 9, 10

On Tuesday, Troy walked into the house as he had predicted, carrying the smell of the diner with him and an old notebook in his hand. He unlaced his boots and pulled them off by the front door before he walked over to the piano. Grace placed a cup of tea with lemon and honey on the table next to the piano, and Troy took his seat on the bench.

They talked about the musical staff, and Grace showed Troy how it works like a graph of time and pitch and can also be viewed something like a map of the keyboard. They talked about the 12 tones, their scales and key signatures and how they fit within the cycle of fifths. As in nature, there are patterns in music, and when you begin to observe them and hear the quality of their characteristics, you can play with them creatively. They talked about rhythmic notation and time signatures and practiced playing rhythms that she wrote on a notebook page for him. Grace wasn't at all surprised that Troy caught on to everything easily. There was a familiarity between his hands and the keyboard like the history shared between old friends.

It had been nearly an hour when Grace noticed the dazed expression of overload in Troy's eyes. "I think that's enough for one sitting, don't you?"

Yawning, he agreed, "Yeah, I think so."

"Give yourself a chance to absorb all of this by practicing and working with it everyday. Practice the scales on your guitar but also on the piano, okay? You seem to have a natural gift for the piano." Grace opened Troy's notebook to a new page and handed it to him. "Here, take this and write down the things you want to work on this week." She gave him a pen so he could come up with his own plan and write it in his own words. Even though it might have seemed like a small act, it was a way for him to take control of what he was learning. As he wrote things down, they talked about ways he could work them into practice. After he made his list, she handed him a beginner's book of piano music. "I'd also like you to take this book home with you and try playing at least one page of music on the piano every day for sightreading practice." Maureen came to mind, and Grace considered how uncomfortable it could be for Troy to practice with her around. "Is there time during the day when you have the house to yourself so you can practice without disturbing anyone?"

"Yeah, there's usually a few hours when everyone's out of the house. I'll practice then." Troy was holding his notebook in his lap, pulling the loose strings of paper through the metal spiral binding. "Grace, remember when you were telling me about how thoughts influence our actions and together they're karmic seeds we plant?"

"Yeah?" She moved away from the piano and sat on the couch to get away from the sunlight that was streaming through the window into her eyes.

"Well, I've been noticing my thoughts more than ever now, and they're not always very good thoughts." He stopped playing with the paper in his notebook and looked up at Grace. "I mean, I really want to have good thoughts and all, but so often I'm really angry." He laughed as if enjoying a private joke with himself. "At least I'm not acting on any of those thoughts." His tone was serious again, "But I can't seem to stop thinking them unless I'm hanging out with my friends, so when I'm home, I just try to stay in my room so I don't have to talk to anyone. I've been reading your book, and there are good things to think about, but trying to do the loving-kindness thing can be really hard."

"But do you see how going into your room so you don't risk acting in anger is a really wise move?" she asked.

Troy agreed, "Yeah, I guess so."

"Whether it's directed at yourself or someone else, anger is destructive. Once the anger is released, its damage is done along with an unfortunate tendency to increase." Grace wanted to show Troy that all things are changeable, including our own perceptions of the people who bring up feelings of anger or hatred. Even though he hadn't named Maureen as the catalyst, she knew he had felt her condemnation. Grace wanted to introduce Troy to the freedom that was within his power—that the nature of everything he encounters requires his cooperation as the perceiver. "You can eliminate anger and its habitual way of showing up in your world by changing your inner world—and by that, I mean your mind." She waited for him to think about what she had just said.

"Well, I kinda understand that from what we talked about the other day. That's why I'm going into my room and closing the door because I know I'm angry. But when someone's always in your face, saying mean things to you, and your own father doesn't stick up for you . . . " His voice tightened, and he cleared his throat to try to push the sadness and the tears away. ". . . and there's nowhere to go . . . " He looked up at the ceiling so tears wouldn't leave his eyes and squeezed his lips tightly together.

Grace sat quietly—breathing as if she could somehow breathe for him and by doing so, soothe the aching in his heart. "Troy, when we're young, parents and other adults hold so much influence over the direction our own lives take. We grow up assuming they're wise and that their conduct and choices will be based on wisdom greater than our own." She looked out the window and watched a blue jay as it hopped from one branch to another on the birch tree outside. "Then, as we grow older, we might realize that they're not the wise souls we trusted them to be—not because they don't want to be, but because they're limited by ignorance." A tear dropped onto the leg of his jeans, and he wiped his eyes with the sleeve of his shirt. "And when I use the word ignorance, I don't mean unintelligent. People can hold degrees from prestigious universities or high positions in government, and even though their brains hold and process lots of knowledge and information, their minds can still be clouded by ignorance." Grace looked down at the floor as if that might give him some privacy for his tears. "Troy, if I had it all figured out with a mind unclouded by ignorance, I'd be so enlightened that I'd be floating over this couch instead of sitting on it." Troy smiled, grateful for her attempt to lighten things up. "But, if you'd like, I'll share some of what I've learned."

Troy cleared his throat where his sadness and frustration were lodged from forcing back tears. "Yeah, please do."

"Based on what you just told me," she began, "I gather life with Maureen has been tough and is one of the challenges that has been tearing you apart lately. Coming out of the semester you just had is uncomfortable enough, but it's salt in an open wound when instead of feeling welcomed home, you're received by hostility."

"Yeah, you got it." His cheeks flushed a wind burned pink.

"I'd like to try to help you shift this experience into something very different," she smiled, "and, if I go off on some tangent that makes no sense, please stop me."

Troy eyed the softer cushions on the green chair and moved from the piano bench to change his seat. "Go for it," he said.

Grace drew in a slow breath, said a silent prayer wishing that her words would benefit and be meaningful for Troy. "Everyone wants happiness. Even though everyone's idea of happiness might be different, all beings—animals included—want whatever their idea of happiness is. But something always seems to throw a wrench in the spokes of happiness because all things change. You change, the weather changes, friends, relationships, the economy, and the planet. Nothing's exempt. Things we think of as permanent and rock solid just aren't fixed in any permanent way. Jobs come and go, wealth can be gained and lost, people who took vows to spend the rest of their lives together end up divorcing, hoping never to see each other again." She rearranged the pillows on the couch, tucking one behind her back and pulling another onto her lap. "But it can go the other way around. For example, someone you couldn't stand in the fifth grade might have been your best friend when you were eighteen. Or countries that once were enemies at war become allies. Keep in mind that none of those examples even take previous lives into account. The Buddhists believe that since beginningless time and over countless lifetimes, all beings could have been your most loved relative *and* your most hated enemy." Even though Troy wasn't sold on the idea, to exclude reincarnation from this conversation would have been like excluding gravity from a discussion on astronomy. "So, between everyone wanting happiness, and everything changing, when people are lucky enough to get the things they believe will make them happy, guess what happens?"

Troy didn't skip a beat. "They get bored, or something goes wrong, or something new comes along that they think is even better." He sat with one ankle crossed over the other knee and was playing with the frayed threads on the hem of his jeans.

"Yes, those happiness-producing things have a limited shelf life, and, eventually, people are unhappy again. Even though we know all things change, people have a visceral dread of it. Thoughts about aging freak us out—just look at how much money people spend buying products and paying for surgeries they believe will spare them from visibly growing older. Out of fear, people cling to other people in relationships. Sometimes people want those relationships to fulfill their own desires to such a degree that they can be downright nasty trying to orchestrate that happening. People cling to possessions and even cling to attitudes and the need to be right. I'm sure you've seen how people can make themselves miserable trying to resist change."

He uncrossed his legs and leaned back in the chair. "I fell apart when my parents got divorced and was a mess wishing they would get back together. When my girlfriend broke up with me, I totally lost it." His thoughts flashed to memories still vividly felt in his heart. "I couldn't concentrate on my classes, didn't care about much of anything, and basically spent the semester drinking and being miserable." He looked at Grace, searching her eyes, hoping she wouldn't judge him for that.

"Troy, it takes time to recover from experiences that cut really deeply into our hearts. So remember that loving-kindness isn't only for everyone else, it's for you too." She adjusted her position on the couch, folding her legs up onto the seat cushion. "And here's some good news—when we understand that change is a good thing, since nothing stays the same, you can take comfort in knowing that if you ever feel you've hit the bottom of your emotional barrel, remember that you won't feel that way forever."

"Ha, that's a good way to look at it." He smiled as if he'd just been let in on a secret that would give him the leverage to pry his way out from the burden of sadness he was under. Or maybe he just got a glimpse of the freedom that exists in change.

Grace went on to explain. "When people are miserable or suffering, Buddhism teaches us that there are three basic causes called the three poisons. Generally they're known as ignorance, desire, and hatred. All three will cause people to do things that make themselves and others even more miserable. With a mind poisoned by hatred and anger, people say cruel things, commit acts of violence, or kill. With a mind poisoned by desire and attachment, people are jealous—they'll steal or destroy. And with a mind poisoned by ignorance—well, we don't have to look very far to see its result. It's an epidemic in the world around us. Ignorance is considered to be the root of the other two, because without ignorance, we're not vulnerable to desire or hatred. Ignorance is like mental blindness that can't see that everyone and everything are interdependent and that one doesn't exist without other.

"Think about how people might treat each other if instead of anger they offered compassion, or if instead of greed they offered generosity. And, instead of seeing

How Generosity Works

life and the world through the eyes of ignorance, what if they were to peel back the murky film of illusion and participate in life with wisdom?"

Troy unbuttoned the cuffs on his flannel shirt and rolled up his sleeves. "It wouldn't be a world any of us would recognize. But it would be awesome if people could get it."

When Troy rolled up his sleeves, Grace realized the house must have been too warm. She reached behind her to open the window. "Well, it begins small. Even one person responding with kindness can make a difference. You know how the pebble toss in the lake works, right? One small circle generates many widening circles radiating out in all directions." She stopped to redirect herself back to Troy's immediate situation. "But, as you were saying, it sounds good, but it's a totally different animal when someone's treating you cruelly, right?" She went into the kitchen and poured Troy a glass of cold apple cider and handed it to him with a napkin and some oatmeal cookies on a small plate.

"Thank you!" He arranged the plate and the glass on the table next to him. "Yes, it is definitely a different animal. I don't know how anyone can really do that. I mean, I know Gandhi did, but he's one guy out of how many billions?" He sipped the cider and set the glass back down on its coaster.

"Well, even if he's one guy out of billions, and even though he's been gone a long time now, the power of what he did is timeless because he's still influencing you and others. Look how immediately he came to your mind to prove it's possible." She enjoyed the way Troy's eyes explored the ceiling when he was considering possibilities.

"Cool. I get it. The ripples from his pebble toss are still here. And come to think of it, Bob Marley and John Lennon, even though they're gone, their music is still rippling out a message of peace and love." Bob Marley and John Lennon were accessible through their music and felt a little closer to home.

"Exactly. So, that tells us never to underestimate the power of one, right? We're moved and inspired by peace, love, and compassion because deep in our hearts we know that's the way it can be and needs to be for everyone. It's not enough to only wish it for ourselves though, because that'll never work." She looked across the room and watched the shadows from the trees' branches moving on the wall while she gathered her thoughts. "It's like if you're in your room all blissed out and tranquil, but in the next room someone starts arguing with someone else, your tranquility is shot to hell, right?"

Troy had finished both cookies and was rubbing the crumbs off his hands onto the legs of his jeans. "Yeah, I guess so. Is that what you meant when you were talking about ignorance being the kind of mind that doesn't recognize the interdependence of everything and everyone?"

"Yes! That's exactly what I meant!" Grace was amazed. He had said it so casually, yet he captured the essence of something immense in its ability to open a different way to perceive obstacles and challenges. She pressed on. "If you see people who are seriously ill or suffering from physical pain, how does that make you feel?"

"Awful. I can't stand to see people in pain. If it's something they're going to heal from like a broken bone, I feel bad, but at least I know they're going to get better." Troy was twisting the paper napkin into spirals around his finger. "But when someone has a chronic or terminal illness and they're in pain, I can't take it. And I feel like an idiot because I can't do a damn thing to help them."

"But you see?" Grace asked. "Your wish would be that you *could* help them, right?"

"Of course. I wish I could help anyone who's sick like that." Since every adult he knew was trying to direct his next step, he immediately added, "Becoming a doctor's not an option though. School and I aren't a good combo. I'd never make it through medical school."

"This isn't about whether or not you're going to be a doctor." She regretted that he thought she was spinning the conversation into career advice. "This is about the strong feeling of compassion you feel when you see someone in pain. The feeling that makes you wish they didn't have to suffer and that you could help them. Even if you're not able to deliver medical care, you *are* able to offer kindness. Loving-kindness goes a long way because it touches the heart.

"People suffer in less obvious ways too. When their minds are clouded by hatred, desire, or ignorance, they are in a different sort of pain. It's a pain that takes hold of their minds and their hearts and delivers them directly to an experience of what could be described as hell. In this case though, we're not talking about a geographical location, we're talking about the way they experience life. When we're on the receiving end of someone consumed by these toxic states of mind, our first reflex is to fight back. But whether we fight back or just seethe in anger, the toxicity has infiltrated our own mind, and the result is that we've jumped into the same hellish sea the other person is drowning in. We might believe we have no choice but to combat anger with anger, and whatever the situation is, that it's out of our control. But the truth is that we are not powerless. We hold enormous power when we understand their behaviors are like the symptoms of a disease. Once we have this understanding, we see their pain and suffering, and instead of responding with anger, we feel compassion just as you do when you see someone with the more obvious outer symptoms of an illness. Remember what we just said about being blissed out in your room and then interrupted by people arguing in the next room?"

"Yup." He finished the last sip of cider. "I might think I have peace, but there is no real peace as long as there are others who are suffering."

His answers were beginning to sound a little too good to be true. "Do you really see that Troy?" Grace asked.

"Yeah, I do. It makes perfect sense." And then with a charming touch of modesty he added, "Don't forget—I've been reading that book, so everything you're saying is tying up some of the loose ends that haven't clicked for me yet."

Grace took Troy's empty glass back into the kitchen to refill it. "Wisdom is the antidote to ignorance, and when you get it, it's like hitting the jackpot at the slot machines," she called out from behind the refrigerator door. "One of the many treasures contained in wisdom is understanding the reality of what you just told me— that because no one and no thing exists by itself, there can be no true peace until all are free from suffering." She brought more cookies and the refreshed glass of cider back to Troy. "So, once you have that understanding, when you see someone who is suffering, your reflexive response becomes compassion. It's like when you have a pain in your foot, your hand instinctively moves to massage and soothe the pain. It's not thinking, 'Oh—that foot has nothing to do with me—I'm a hand, and I'm not in pain, so let that foot just deal with its own pain. Its pain is not my problem.' With wisdom, we understand that all beings are connected through causes and conditions. We understand that we're all part of the same karmic results. We have the choice to stop the vicious cycle of pain and suffering by generating good actions that bring good karmic results instead. When our minds are infused with wisdom, we will have the impulse to relieve pain for others just like the hand has for the foot. Then, when we thoroughly and unshakably comprehend that we are all connected—that there is no real separation between one and another—we will have uncovered the alchemic power to convert disharmony into peace. This alchemic power is the spirit of enlightenment or bodhicitta mind."

The sun slipped behind the trees in the distance and sent light filtering through their branches, splashing off the frosted rooftops and windowpanes on the houses that nested in the hills. It was that time of day when winter afternoons turn the sky from blue to a bruised shade of purple. A cold draft of air blew through the open window behind Grace. She stood to close the window and then to switch the lamps on. The coldness in the room reminded her that the fire needed attention. "Troy, I hope I haven't overwhelmed you with way more than you wanted to hear about." She walked down the stairs to tend the fire.

"Not at all. From the moment I picked up that book the first day I came here, I knew I wanted to understand more." Grace was surprised to hear Troy's voice close behind her and that he had followed her down the stairs.

"Do you want some help with that?" he offered.

Accustomed to doing everything by herself, she was already crouched down by the wood stove, adding newspaper and arranging the new pieces of wood into the flames. "Thanks, Troy, but I've got it."

"It looks as if you could use some more wood though. I'll bring some in for you. Where do you keep it?" He was already by the front door putting his boots and gloves on.

"That would be wonderful. Thank you." The independence that kept her strong was the same independence that made it awkward for her to accept help. Knowing that it was important for Troy to have his kindness received, she resisted her first impulse to decline his offer. "I keep it out in the back corner of the yard by the fence. I'll go turn the lights on in the back for you." And as she switched on the outdoor lights she told him, "There's a plastic toboggan near the woodpile that you can use to haul the wood back to the house."

While Troy was getting the wood, Grace took the dishes back into the kitchen. Troy came in and out of the house several times carrying armloads of wood that he carefully stacked by the wall for her. It was enough wood to keep the fire going for the rest of the week. Grace had written some instructions for meditation to give him. She explained that among other benefits, meditation is a way we can prepare ourselves for handling obstacles such as his relationship with Maureen. Rinpoche had said that meditation is the way to firmly etch in our hearts and minds the lessons learned from study, teachings, and contemplation. Through the practice gained during meditation, when we encounter challenges in our daily life, we will more likely respond with compassion instead of anger or self-pity.

"Troy, thank you so much for carrying all that wood in for me." His face was flushed from the cold air outside. He stood by the door so he wouldn't have to take his boots off again, and Grace handed him his notebook, music, and a container filled with the rest of the oatmeal cookies. "I guess I'll either see you on Thursday with Natalie or next Tuesday at three o'clock?"

"Or maybe both," he answered. "I loved the music lesson, our conversation, and all you taught me today. Thank you. I've got lots to practice." He opened the door to leave. "See you soon."

Part Two

Practice

May a rain of food and drink descend
To clear away the pain of thirst and hunger,
And during the aeon of famine
May I myself change into food and drink.
III. v. 9

The windows on Troy's truck were sealed under a thin layer of ice. When he climbed in, the coldness of the seats and steering wheel penetrated through his clothes. He turned the key in the ignition, and the engine turned over and then quickly sputtered off again. After two more attempts and a little extra gas with the last turn of the key, the engine was running. Troy blasted the heat and the defroster that sent out cold air until the engine was warm. He rummaged through the empty soda cans and fast-food bags on the floor of the truck to find the snow brush with an ice scraper on its handle that had fallen between the seat and the door. Before he quit smoking, this would have been his cue to light up and take a cigarette outside with him to clear the windows. It had been over six months since he quit, but there were still moments that provoked the craving to smoke. After the discussion with Grace, he understood the deceptive side to desire, and, instead of being tormented by the craving, it left him almost as quickly as it came. The defroster began to melt the ice on the front windshield while he scraped the ice off the side and back windows. The truck was warmer when he climbed back in, and he settled comfortably into his seat.

He wasn't in a rush to get home, so he took the slower route through town instead of the back roads. Waiting at a stoplight, he saw a man in an old wool coat pushing a grocery cart filled with bottles and cans heading in the direction of the package store on the corner. There were redemption machines outside the store where people could return their empty bottles for cash. Resigned to the cold, the man walked slowly, watching his feet as if he needed reassurance to see that they knew where they were going. He wore a wide rimmed leather hat and a long knit scarf coiled around his neck up to his ears. Troy watched him while he was waiting for the light to turn until he felt the uncomfortable pang of sadness that comes when you see someone whose life is a harsh struggle for survival. It was a combination of frustration and shame that made him look away. His eyes lowered to the mess of empty cans in his truck, and he had what he thought was a brilliant idea. When the light changed, he turned and drove ahead of the man to the package store. Troy

How Generosity Works

gathered all the cans that had accumulated over the past several weeks and stuffed them into the bags that had fallen on the floor. On the passenger seat, there was a sandwich he had brought from work and the cookies Grace had given him. Troy put them out along with the cans, moving with the speed and focus of an emergency drill. He arranged everything in a pile by the machines and, before he left, reached into his jeans pocket and pulled out eighteen dollars he had earned in tips and weighted the money under the sandwich. He drove out of the parking lot as the man made his way to the redemption area and pulled over to the side of the road to watch him find the collection waiting for him. The man stood in his oversized grey wool coat under the store's spotlights and looked around to see if anyone else was nearby. He picked up the sandwich, cookies and cash, put them in his coat pockets, and began feeding the bottles and cans into the machines.

Troy continued on through town, inching along with the other cars that were sifting through the string of traffic lights over every intersection. He imagined the man savoring each bite of the sandwich and cookies, and buying something special with the extra cash. He hoped there was a shelter where he would find warmth.

If, in those who encounter me,
A faithful or an angry thought arises,
May that eternally become the source
For fulfilling all their wishes.

May all who say bad things to me
Or cause me any other harm,
and those who mock and insult me
Have the fortune to fully awaken.
III. v. 16, 17

Emerging on the other side of town, the road wound past homes spaced far apart on landscaped properties that, in the lush green days of summer, look like advertisements in a lawn products catalog. Troy pulled into the long driveway that circled in front of his father's and Maureen's house and parked in the corner of the driveway near the snow-bank where the plow had piled the snow. He walked up the flagstone path to the front entrance and into the foyer with the pretentiously high ceiling and giant chandelier dangling overhead. He walked past the marble-topped mahogany table, up the stairs that curved in a spiral around the chandelier to the second floor, down the long hallway towards the back of the house, and into his room. Closing the door behind him, he tossed his books onto his bed and took off his boots. His father, Maureen, and Natalie were downstairs having dinner. He was hungry and wanted to join them, but the thought of sitting with Maureen and her sideways technique of watching him and then rolling her eyes at his father tangled his stomach into knots. He sat on the edge of his bed, closed his eyes and breathed. That's all he did for about five minutes. Then, he opened his eyes, stood and, opened the door to go downstairs.

His footsteps were silent on the thickly carpeted floor in the living room. He could hear the sound of silverware on plates and his father and Maureen talking in the kitchen.

Natalie saw him first, "Troy's here!" She slid off her chair, ran toward him, and jumped for him to pick her up.

"Hey, Nat!" He caught her in his arms, gave her a squeeze, and carried her back over to her seat at the table.

"Hi, Maureen," he said. Maureen didn't look up; she was carving the steak on her plate. Troy leaned over to hug his father on the way to his seat, "Hi, Dad."

Maureen didn't take her eyes off her steak when she spoke to Troy, "Don't call her Nat. Gnats are annoying insects. Her name is Natalie." She shot a piercing look at Brian that was more lethal than the knife she held in her hand.

Troy said, "I'm sorry. I never thought of it like that before." He helped himself to salad and to a portion of ziti with marinara sauce. "Natalie, please pass the parmesan cheese."

Natalie handed him the small bowl with the grated parmesan cheese and the spoon to serve it with.

"Where have you been?" Brian asked. He had a habit of wiping his mouth with his napkin every time he spoke.

"After work today, I had a music lesson from Natalie's piano teacher. I want to learn how to read music and about scales and chords. It'll help me with the guitar."

"Who's paying for that?" Maureen asked.

"I am." Troy answered. The truth was, he and Grace hadn't discussed money. It was something he'd need to ask her about next time he saw her. He changed the subject. "The ziti's delicious, Maureen."

Maureen held her fork midway between her plate and her mouth and with her eyes still on her plate said, "Thanks."

Brian took a bite of salad. "Natalie sounds good on the piano," chewing between his words, "so that lady must be a good teacher." He didn't just dab at the corners of his mouth with his napkin, it was more like he was mopping up a large spill on his face.

"Daddy, I'm learning a new song. Do you want to hear it?" Natalie was off the chair before she finished asking.

"After dinner, Natalie. Get back in your seat," he answered.

She settled back into her chair, and Maureen put a piece of steak on her fork for her. She held the fork, coaxing Natalie to eat more. "She's a decent teacher, but what's up with her? I mean, she just lives in that house all by herself. She doesn't have a husband or even a boyfriend. I think there must be something wrong with her."

Troy wanted to defend Grace but didn't want to instigate another attack. "I'm pretty sure she was married before. She's got a couple of kids she talks about who are already grown up. Maybe marriage was just a really bad experience for her."

"Maybe she's just old and ugly!" Brian laughed from behind his napkin.

"She is not!" Natalie wailed. "She's really pretty and really nice, and I love her."

Brian lowered his voice, "Sorry, Natalie. I was just joking." The apology was too late because Natalie had already begun to cry.

"Don't cry." Maureen reached her arm around Natalie's shoulder and brought her closer to herself. "We know Grace is a nice lady or we wouldn't let you take piano lessons from her." She rolled her eyes at Brian and mouthed "asshole" at him.

Everyone had finished their dinner except Natalie. Brian kept eating, whether he was hungry or not, as long as there was food within reach.

Troy looked at Natalie. "If you finish your dinner, I'll clean up while you play your new song for Maureen and Dad."

Natalie hurried to finish the rest of the ziti and most of her salad. "Okay. I'm finished. Come on, let's go."

She ran ahead into the living room while Brian grabbed one more piece of garlic bread and ate it, dropping crumbs, as he walked behind her. Maureen started clearing the table and carrying dishes over to the sink.

"Maureen, go enjoy Natalie's song and relax. I'll take care of the dishes." Troy opened the dishwasher and began rinsing the plates before loading them.

It was hard for Maureen to relinquish control of her kitchen to anyone, but especially to Troy. And she didn't like him instructing her to relax. She pulled containers out from the cupboard. "Here, Troy, use these for the leftovers. Just put water in the pots to soak, I'll wash them later." She took the spray cleanser out from under the sink and handed him the sponge she used for countertops. "Use this to wipe down the table and the counters, and don't forget the front of the refrigerator and the stove and around the burners."

"Okay."

Natalie yelled from the other room, "Mommy, come on! We're waiting for you!"

As she was leaving the kitchen, Troy said, "Thank you for dinner. It was delicious."

Maureen was out of the room, stopped walking, and then without looking back muttered, "You're welcome," and continued into the living room.

Brian was sitting on the big yellow and white brocade sofa with his arms stretched across the top and motioned for Maureen to sit next to him. As she sat down, she leaned toward Brian and whispered, "What the hell's going on with Troy? He's acting weird."

Brian shrugged his shoulders and whispered back, "Maybe he's just happy."

Maureen was still not satisfied. "I think Grace used to be a hippie. Do you think she gave him drugs?"

A man of few words, Brian answered, "No."

Natalie was at the piano with her music open, hands resting on the keys ready to play. "This is a minuet by Mozart." She began playing while Maureen and Brian sat closer together than they'd been in ages. It took a minute, but Maureen relaxed and melted into the comfort of feeling Brian's arm around her and closed her eyes to listen to Natalie's playing.

⌐

Leisure and endowment are very hard to find;
And, since they accomplish what is meaningful for
humanity,
If I do not take advantage of them now,
How will such a perfect opportunity come about
again?
I. v. 4

The alarm clock blared viciously loud and out of tune chimes, jolting Troy from sleep at four o'clock Wednesday morning. Opening his eyes to a room that was still too dark for shadows, he dug through his mind to remember what in God's name he was doing awake at this hour. Slowly, the reasons came sifting back into his mind. He needed to be at work by five-thirty to set up for breakfast customers. And he wanted to see if meditating in the morning would really make a difference. Grace had explained that our minds are the most open and fresh when we first wake up. She said the mind is like newly fallen snow before any footprints have left their mark, because it hasn't yet been invaded by the busy and more frantic habits of thought. She had also told him that declaring your intentions for the new day when you first open your eyes is a powerful practice. "Each day provides material to expand your mind into wisdom," she had said. "Setting your motivation is a way of greeting the day and welcoming the conditions it presents—which, don't forget, are all karmically generated."

Thinking of the things he and Grace had talked about the day before, Troy began to formulate his intention silently in his mind. *All my thoughts, words, and actions will be filled with loving-kindness and compassion, with equanimity for the sake of all living beings.* He repeated these intentions several times and then turned on the light by his bed to read something Grace had written on an index card for him:

Conquer the angry man by love.
Conquer the ill-natured man by goodness.
Conquer the miser with generosity.
Conquer the liar with truth.
[The Buddha, "The Dhammapada"]

As he reflected on those words, he thought, *maybe the man this is referring to could be either myself or someone else. Even if I don't conquer Maureen's anger, at least I can conquer my own.*

After he washed up and dressed, he got ready to practice the meditation that Grace had taught him. He folded his blanket into a small square to use as a cushion and sat on the floor with his legs crossed and his spine straight. That seemed easy enough to do. His arms were loose, elbows slightly bent, his hands resting comfortably on his lap and against his lower abdomen. He nested the back of his right hand within the open palm of his left with his thumbs lightly touching each other and pointing up towards the ceiling the way

Grace had shown him. His eyes were closed, his lips slightly parted, and the tip of his tongue touched the roof of his mouth just behind his teeth. He brought his attention to his breath. Grace had told him simply to notice the breath going out and coming in again. As thoughts came up, she had said not to judge them or entertain them, but to imagine them like fish-bubbles, bubbling up and floating away. "Release them," she had said, "and then gently bring the attention back to the breath. The breath is always with us, so we have a perfect object to focus on that lets us practice anytime and anywhere."

Keeping his mind on his breathing was harder than he'd expected. His mind chased random thoughts that entered from every whichway. Even though Grace had told him this might happen, he was feeling discouraged. He tried again and managed to follow three breaths before becoming distracted again. *I wonder how that guy liked the sandwich I left for him? I wonder where he slept last night?*

Troy sat in this meditation for not quite ten minutes, and it went back and forth like this with small exchanges between focus and distraction. Overall, he felt calm even up to the point when his legs started to hurt and his foot fell asleep.

Opening his eyes, he stood up, shook his legs out, grabbed his coat and keys, and walked as quietly as he could downstairs and out the door.

The moon, just a few days away from being full, was setting low in the horizon. The sky had the serenity of twilight as the last of the night's stars were fading from sight. Troy smelled sweetness in the air from the row of white pines that bordered the driveway and stood outside his truck soaking in the scents of dawn.

It took a few tries before the engine turned over. Troy let it idle for a few minutes before he put it in reverse and backed out the long driveway to the street. Winding his way through the neighborhood roads into town, he drove past the building where he had gone to school—the place where he first lost interest in learning. Then, past the frozen river where he and his friends used to hide—skipping classes and smoking cigarettes. It was on the banks of this river, sheltered under the cover of trees, that they shared their dreams for the freedom they imagined on the other side of childhood. He passed the hill where he and his best friend climbed one day to sit on a rock and spent the afternoon talking and laughing in the sun. It was the last time he saw Jason before he was killed. A speeding driver had hit him while he was walking home one night. Troy was glad the memories were of laughter, but they still brought a flood of tears to his eyes and a pain that he discovered no amount of drinking would take away. He had seen first hand that life is precious and fleeting. He had also come to understand that when he is ready to pay attention, life teaches him what he needs to learn. He was paying attention now.

The morning moved fast through the breakfast shift. People poured in for takeout orders while others sat in their regular seats at the counter. The counter was where the daily customers sat, greeting each other like extended family. The tables were where people sat to discuss business, and, later in the morning, the mothers who had dropped their children off at school would meet to chat—their smaller children strapped into high chairs. Troy liked the fast pace of the diner. Bussing tables and setting them for the next customers were his tasks, and he did them well.

Hours had passed like minutes when the breakfast crowd cleared, and Troy was wiping down the table by the front window. Watching the activity of people passing by, he saw the man with the grocery cart picking up an empty can that someone had thrown onto the street. He left the rag on the table and ran into the kitchen where he filled a cardboard container with chili and rice and put it in a bag with a plastic spoon, napkins, crackers, and a can of apple juice.

"I'll be right back," he told the cook who was sitting on a stool holding a cup of coffee, resting from the morning rush.

Troy didn't have to run far to catch up to the man who had moved on to the garbage can near the library. He was looking loosely through the garbage for bottles to add to his collection.

"Excuse me," Troy said as he approached the man. Now that he was up close, he could see the man's eyes were sky blue. Squinting into the sun, there was a distance in his eyes that looked back at Troy as if he had just intruded into another world. "Here's some hot chili and rice," Troy said as he handed the bag to the man. He wanted to say more, but he was caught off guard by the power behind those eyes and at a loss for words except to say, "Have a good day." He turned and walked back to the diner where Maggie, the waitress, stood watching through the glass door and greeted him with her smile that had the ability to turn him inside out. He had temporarily lost the capacity to speak, so he flickered a smile and picked up the rag where he had left it and finished wiping down the tables and set up for lunch.

The lunch shift passed a little more slowly than breakfast had with a sparser flow of customers. Those who came for lunch lingered in conversation, drinking coffee, and eating pieces of pecan or apple pie. When their plates were empty, they absentmindedly curled the edges of their paper place mats while they talked. Another storm was on its way later in the evening, and already the sky was beginning to thicken with clouds. Everyone was speculating on how much snow would fall; estimates were between six and ten inches.

Troy cleared dishes from customers' tables while Maggie filled coffee cups and unloaded fistfuls of little plastic creamers into the centers of the tables. He could feel the weight of Maggie watching him as the afternoon went on. When they passed each other, circling from table to table, he returned her smiles, making his best effort to act nonchalant. Considering she was the prettiest girl he had ever seen, pulling off casually cool was a challenge.

Just breathe, he told himself. *You're getting all attached and freaked out about stuff you're only imagining. Just enjoy the moment, that's all.*

Nervousness dissipated when everything rearranged itself in his mind. Maggie was no different from himself or the man pushing the grocery cart through town—she wanted what everyone wants—just to be happy. A rush of compassion shook everything upside down and right side up into perfect order when he realized that he desired happiness for Maggie more than he desired her, or anything for himself.

"Are you working tomorrow?" Maggie asked Troy as they were putting their coats on to leave.

"No. I have tomorrow off," he said. "I'll be in on Friday though. What about you?"

"I'll be here," she said.

"If it's a nice day, do you want to take a walk in the woods after work?" he asked. "It's always really beautiful in there after the snow." Whether she accepted the invitation or not wasn't a deal breaker for his day falling apart or holding together. But he did hope she would say yes.

"I'd love to," she said.

⌣

What then be said then of one
Who eternally bestows the peerless bliss of the Sugatas
Upon limitless numbers of beings,
Thereby fulfilling all their hopes?

However, if a virtuous attitude should arise (in that
regard),
Its fruits will multiply far more than that,
When Bodhisattvas greatly suffer they generate no
negativity,
Instead their virtues naturally increase.
I. v. 33, 35

There was no one home when Troy got back to the house, and he felt a welcoming relief in its emptiness. He saw the pieces of mail that Maureen had tossed onto his unmade bed, scattered as if by a turbulent wind. Sorting through them would wait until later. A shower and clean clothes took priority.

Troy stood in the shower's steam, reflecting on all that had happened since he left Grace's house the day before. If someone had asked him to describe what was different, it would have been a struggle to find the words. To an objective observer, there was no change in circumstances. But for Troy, there was an inner bubbling of excitement like setting off on a road trip to visit someplace he'd never been before. He might have described it as the sense of freedom that comes when you load your car with only the things you really need, leaving your routines and worries behind. And then, once on your way, the sweetness that envelops you when you open the windows to breathe the air and take in the new scenery. He knew there could be setbacks like traffic jams or construction that would slow him down and dampen his enthusiasm. But he felt a sense of certainty that the road he was on was taking him someplace he wanted to go.

When he remembered that one of those potential setbacks, in the form of Maureen, would cross his path soon, his peace turned to panic. She would be bringing Natalie home from school in less than an hour. Troy turned off the water, dried off, and got dressed. He filled his arms with dirty clothes that were piled on his bedroom floor, ran downstairs to the laundry room, threw the clothes and a capful of detergent into the washing machine, and started the machine running. His heart was racing when he stopped where he was in the hallway outside the laundry room. "I'm not doing this anymore." He actually spoke the words out loud. His happy little roadtrip had just taken him to an intersection of insight where he recognized that the way he thought of Maureen had circled him right back to the place he'd left behind. With that insight, he understood fully what Grace meant when she was talking about the people arguing in the next room interrupting his peace. In Troy's world, Maureen was the miserable person in the next room, and until she was happy, there could be no peace. Until he could offer her compassion with the same generosity he would a stranger—like the man in town—or a close friend, ignorance would run the show. He knew what was needed, but he didn't know if he had the confidence or the strength to pull it off. He recalled Grace explaining that this is one reason why people practice meditation. It provides a mental dress rehearsal to prepare us for the head-on experiences that strike in daily life.

Back in his room, he picked up the book Grace had given him. He had turned down corners of certain pages to mark places he wanted to refer to again. He found the page he was looking for and read the segment about equanimity and referred to Grace's instructions on how to practice it in meditation. It involved a lot of imagination, stretching it in ways he wasn't accustomed to. Grace had told him these things would become easier for him with focused effort and practice.

He took his seat on the makeshift cushion he had left on the floor in front of his bedroom windows. Looking across the field, he could see a stretch of woods that divided his neighborhood from the others that were closer to town. The variety of trees crowding together, their limbs bare for the winter and reaching into all corners of the sky, reflected the afternoon sun filtering through the clouds like a study in light and texture. Troy watched the squirrels chase each other over the maze of branches, appearing to defy gravity as they ran from one tree to another. Then, he closed his eyes and shifted his awareness to the feeling of his breath entering and leaving his body. He imagined his mind as the sky and his thoughts as clouds floating past on a slow, steady breeze until the sky grew quite clear. He had the sense of himself being inseparable from the sky and breathed into that feeling of oneness.

He began to contemplate karma and how all things—every thought, every action, and every encounter—are the result of causes and conditions. He sat with that for a while to consider how it played out in his own life, in world events, and even environmental concerns for the planet. His thoughts began to wander a bit so he brought his attention back to his breath, breathing in that sense of oneness.

With the awareness that all beings have the common desire to be happy and to be free of suffering, he then proceeded into another layer of meditation known as analytical meditation. First, he needed to think about someone he felt a genuine and uncomplicated love towards. An image of Natalie automatically came to his mind. It was easy to feel warmth and love with thoughts of her. The analytical portion of the meditation involved examining where all those wonderful and warm feelings came from. The causes and conditions that brought Natalie and him into each other's lives could have been entirely different. What if Natalie had been a distant neighbor at the end of the block who he barely knew? The true cause of the warmth he felt towards Natalie wasn't Natalie, but the love itself. The love, like everything that manifests in life, was the result of the ongoing chain of causes and conditions.

The next step in this particular meditation was to bring to mind someone he didn't know well, someone for whom his feelings were neutral. It could have been a person he'd seen while sitting in a line of traffic, the cashier at the gas station, or one of the customers at the diner. There was no special affection or dislike for this person due to the absence of causes and conditions to create either feeling. And that's the point. The person alone is not the container of the feelings as if he or she is inherently bad or inherently good. For example, if one day he were to be driving down the road and had a flat tire and this particular person were to pull over to help change it, he'd consider that person to be good, and be filled with gratitude. But, if instead the same person smashed into his car, he'd consider that person to be bad and would be filled with aggravation. Again, it is causes and conditions that would have created either feeling. According to the Buddhist teachings, in any of our previous lifetimes, all beings could have been our precious mother who took care of us and without whom we would never have survived. In this meditation, Troy imagined this neutral person as having been a loving mother and thought about the kindness she would have cared for him with. The same feeling of warmth and love he spontaneously felt for Natalie began to arise for this neutral person. He sat with this feeling for a few minutes, dissolving into the sense of oneness he had felt earlier.

Finally, it was time to think of someone who brought up feelings of anger. As fast as Maureen popped into his mind, so did the urge to push her away. Instead, he held her in his mind, breathed, and dived more deeply into the analytical meditation. He contemplated that there must have been conditions in Maureen's life that caused her to behave as she did.

If her mind were at peace she wouldn't snap at Troy like a walking, spring-loaded trap of hostility. The three poisons, as Grace had explained, were the causes and conditions that influenced Maureen's actions. As he had done with the neutral person, he recognized that Maureen by herself was not the container for his unpleasant feelings. How could she be when his father thought she was the love of his life? Maureen by herself, without other causes and conditions, could not be the sole source of his misery or his father's joy.

Recognizing that it is causes and conditions that create negative and positive feelings, not just one person or one thing existing by itself, he then plunged more deeply into the meditation. He applied the same analytical practice he had used when thinking about the neutral person. He imagined that at another time, under different circumstances, Maureen could have been someone who was very kind to him. For a moment, he actually had a feeling of love for her and a strong sense of wanting her to experience happiness.

The fact that he felt this way about Maureen caught him by surprise and distracted him. He had to work to bring his mind back to continue in the meditation and back into the feeling of love and equanimity. He determined that he wanted to overcome the causes and conditions within his own mind that create negative feelings. He made a promise to himself that he would hold the understandings he had arrived at during this meditation in his mind and let them guide his own actions. He then made a wish for all beings to have the causes and conditions for happiness and the causes and conditions to be free of suffering. Returning his focus to the awareness of his breath, and then to the sensations of his body, he opened his eyes.

Hoping that his clothes had finished washing, he walked downstairs to the laundry room. The washing machine had just clicked past the end of its cycle, still shaking from its last spin. He opened the lid to pull the wet clothes out and was putting them into the dryer when he heard the garage door open. He started the dryer running and walked into the kitchen to open the door for Maureen and Natalie.

Natalie was already out of the car, dragging her book bag along the floor by its strap. Maureen was getting groceries from the back.

"Hi," Troy said, "I'll help you with those bags." He walked over to the car to help carry the groceries into the house. Looping the handles of several bags onto each hand, he was able to carry all the remaining bags at once.

Natalie watched him lift all the bags together onto the counter. Her eyes wide, she was convinced that this was all the proof necessary to declare that she, in fact, had the strongest brother of all her friends. She threw her arms around him and hugged him like she'd never let him go.

Maureen was putting the groceries away, emptying the bags as if she were trying to set a record for speed. She was rearranging the shelves in the refrigerator to make room for a package of chicken. When she lifted one of the containers Troy had filled the night before, the top came off and the leftover ziti poured onto the floor. She screamed, "Goddamnit, Troy!" She glared at him as she whisked past him to grab some paper towels. "You piece of shit, can't you do *anything* right?" She began mopping up the floor.

Troy pulled a few sheets of paper towels off the roll, wet them with cold water, and bent down to help. "I'm so sorry," he said. "I'll clean it up." He looked at Maureen and saw her face was contorted by rage. But he didn't just see her as a woman in a fit of anger, he saw her as someone suffering from a mind consumed by hatred. He felt a deep compassion for her as he would for someone with a terminal illness who was suffering intense physical pain. He finished cleaning the ziti from the floor while Maureen put groceries away, throwing cupboard doors open and slamming them shut.

"Troy didn't do it, Mommy." Natalie leaped to her brother's defense. "I saw Daddy eating from that last night after you listened to my song."

"I don't want to hear it, Natalie." Maureen was not one to be corrected. "You stay out of this. Take your book bag to your room and get started on your homework."

Troy remembered something he had read that portrayed the senselessness of being angry at the person who mistreats you. It was an allegorical illustration that pointed out that if someone hits you with a stick, it's not the stick you are angry with. It's important to understand that it is the poisoned mind that causes a person to lash out, generating more negative karma in their wake. Maureen was consumed by anger that was essentially choking the life out of herself and sending her further into a miserable existence.

Troy was silent while he used cleanser to wipe the marinara sauce from the white tile. He drew on the strength from his meditation and applied compassion to Maureen's anger, treating it with the tenderness he would an open wound. To his amazement, she appeared to him as someone he loved and who he wanted to help. He finished cleaning the floor and opened the cupboard under the sink to toss the used paper towels into the garbage.

"I'm sorry, Troy," Maureen spoke, her voice softer than he'd ever heard it. "I'm really sorry," she said again, this time her voice was almost a whisper.

Troy looked at her. She wasn't looking back at him. She was standing in front of the cabinets, with her hands resting on the counter, looking at the patterns on the granite countertop.

"I was totally out of line with what I said just now." She reached for the paper towels again, this time to blot her eyes. "But it's not only for this that I'm apologizing." Her voice rose a little higher, and she began to sob. "The way I've treated you since you've been home has been so wretched that I can't even stand myself anymore." The sobbing swelled into anguished, painful moans. She took several sheets of paper towels off the roll and pressed them against her face. "I don't know what's the matter with me or why I've got it in my head that I'm supposed to hate you when really, you're just a guy trying to do everything you can to make your life better."

Troy couldn't believe what he was hearing. The entire encounter felt like an out-of-body experience.

Maybe that's exactly what had happened—maybe they had broken through their labeled containers of good guy and bad guy and now were just two people experiencing causes and conditions. He wasn't sure what to say or do. In fact, he wished he didn't have to say anything at all, but he felt Maureen deserved an acknowledgement for her apology. "Thanks, Maureen," he said. "I'm sorry it's been so hard." He didn't have anything more profound than that to say, although he thought he should have been able to do better than *thanks* and *I'm sorry it's been so hard*. But he had spoken from his heart, as simple as it might have been.

"Well, it doesn't need to be hard at all." Maureen looked at Troy, her mascara had washed into dark smudges under her eyes. "Sometimes I'm just slow to catch onto things." She looked away again and over at the two bags of groceries that hadn't been emptied yet.

She began putting groceries away again. "I'll start dinner. Would you go check on Natalie and see if she needs any help with her homework?"

"Sure," he said. But the room held a trance-like balance, and Troy feared that even taking a step in the direction out of the room risked throwing it all back into the crazy windstorm of a few minutes earlier. And then he saw how fast his thoughts ran to the wrong perception. The kind of thinking that believes something exists in a concrete and isolated way had immediately walloped him with fear. He smiled at the powerful simplicity of what had just taken place and the new causes and conditions that had developed as a result. He smiled at Maureen who was still wiping tears from her eyes and said, "I'll go check on Natalie."

All other virtues are like plantain trees;
For after bearing fruit, they simply perish.
Yet the perennial tree of the Awakening Mind
Unceasingly bears fruit and thereby flourishes without
end.

Just like the fire at the end of an age,
It instantly consumes all great wrongdoing,
Its unfathomable advantages were taught
to the disciple Sudhana by the wise Lord Maitreya.
I. v. 12, 14

When Troy got to Natalie's room, her door was closed. He knocked on the door, "Natalie—hey, can I come in?"

"Yeah," she answered.

When he opened the door, she was sitting on the floor with her dolls, dressing them for an outing. One doll was already in a small pink convertible, dressed complete with hat and fur coat, one arm extended as if waving. The other doll, arms raised straight up, was having a gold lamé evening gown pulled over its head.

"Hi, Nat," Troy said as he sat down on the floor opposite her and the assembly of dolls and wardrobe. "Do you need any help with your homework?"

"No," she said, her face straining with concentration as she struggled to pull the gown over her doll's torso smoothly. "I did it already." With the dress on the doll, she began searching the collection of accessories. She picked up a tiny turquoise boa and wrapped it around the doll's shoulders. "Why is Mommy so mean?" she asked.

"She was pretty angry, wasn't she?" Troy laughed to lighten things up for her. "That's what happens when people get angry, but she's better now."

Natalie found a pink belt that she put around the doll's waist and then searched through the assortment of miniscule plastic shoes to find a matching pair. "I hope I never get angry like that."

"You probably won't," Troy reassured her. "Your doll looks gorgeous. Where's she going?"

"Well, you see," she began with a very serious tone, "first they're going for a very long drive, and then they're going dancing." She held the doll up by its ankles and twisted it a little from side to side to check the outfit. She then held the doll out for Troy's inspection. "Do you think she needs earrings?"

"Try some on her and see how they look," he answered.

Now on the hunt for earrings, she asked, "Will you take me to my piano lesson tomorrow?"

"I'd love to," he said. He thought about all the things he wanted to tell Grace. But maybe, he thought, she already knows.

⌐

The Awakening Mind is the supreme medicine
That quells the world's diseases.
It is the tree that shelters all beings
Wandering and tired on the path of conditioned
existence.

It is the universal bridge
That leads to freedom from unhappy states of birth,
It is the dawning moon of the mind
That dispels the torment of disturbing conceptions.

It is the great sun that finally removes
The misty ignorance of the world,
It is the quintessential butter
From the churning of the milk of Dharma.

For all those guests traveling on the path of
conditioned existence
Who wish to experience the bounties of happiness,
This will satisfy them with joy
And actually place them in supreme bliss.
III. v. 30, 31, 32, 33

Acknowledgments

It was the vision and guiding wisdom of John Cerullo at Diamond Cutter Press that made this book possible, along with Casey Kemp's skillful editing that held all material accountable to the Dharma and Clare Cerullo's thoughtful finetuning, layout, and design.

I am forever grateful to my sons, Geoffrey and Daniel, for filling my life with joy, inspiration, and love.